The **Body** **Shape** *Diet*

Your hands, face, and figure tell all
about how you can improve
your metabolism, nutrition,
and hormonal status.

Dr. Cass Ingram

KNOWLEDGE
HOUSE
PUBLISHERS

First Edition, formerly published as *Eat Right 4 Your Metabolic Type*

Printed in the United States of America

ISBN: 978-1-931078-28-3

Disclaimer: This book is not intended as a substitute for medical diagnosis or treatment. Anyone who has a serious disease should consult a physician before initiating any change in treatment or before beginning any new treatment.

To order this or additional Knowledge House books call: 1-866-626-5888 or order via the web at: www.knowledgehousepublishers.com

To get an order form send a SASE to:
Knowledge House Publishers
105 East Townline Rd., Unit 116
Vernon Hills, IL 60061

The
Body
Shape
Diet

Table of Contents

Dedication

For those who desire perfect health

Introduction

There is a simple tool for improving overall health. It is based upon a person's shape. Thus, it is easy to understand. It is also easy to apply. In fact, it is so simple that anyone can immediately gain the benefits. Regardless of race, culture, or background everyone can benefit from this system. It is a key, even a secret, to a longer and fuller life.

The body is like a book to be read. It reveals its secrets—a kind of code that tells all. This is the secret code of the hormone system. Here, this code is broken and the secret revealed. It is revealed mainly by a person's shape. The shape tells the state of a person's endocrine system and how it affects his or her metabolism. This is known as the endocrine or hormonal type. Then, this type serves as a guide to therapy, because the hormone system controls all. With the proper therapy the health improves rapidly. This is achieved specifically through discovering the endocrine body type and prescribing the appropriate treatment. The endocrine type and the metabolic type are synonymous. The endocrine system is essentially the hormone system. It is that system of glands which produces the various hormones. What's more, hormones control and influence all cell functions.

There are four main metabolic/endocrine types. These are the primary endocrine body types. There are two additional types, which are more rare. These are the secondary or ancillary types. This book emphasizes the four main types.

Each person can learn how to determine his or her type. This is critical. This is because the endocrine type guides the appropriate therapy. With the correct assessment, with the right diagnosis, then, the correct and accurate approach can be taken. Then, the person would expect to gain powerful results, which is to achieve the greatest health possible. It is also so that the person can remain in ideal health, since the endocrine type is the tool for the prevention of major diseases.

There is an obvious reason to be concerned about the health of Western people. Such people lead the world in degenerative diseases. The majority of such diseases are related to glandular function. In other words, the glands are functioning abnormally, which precipitates disease.

Again, the health of Western people is in decline. In this decline the endocrine system plays a monumental role. This is based upon first-hand observations. After giving hundreds of lectures and seminars, as well as countless radio/TV appearances, one issue is clear. There are hidden epidemics occurring throughout Western countries. These are related to more than just germs or cancer. In fact, these epidemics are metabolic disorders, which are equally as devastating as infections. Plus, these disorders are directly due to wrong diet.

The majority of people have endocrine disorders. This is especially true for people living under mental stress as well as those who suffer from poor nutrition. This means that the majority of Westerners, that is Americans, Canadians, and Europeans, have defective metabolism. Without treatment, the consequences are often dire: ill health, obesity, and outright disease, including killer diseases such as arthritis, diabetes, heart disease, high blood pressure, kidney disease, lupus, immune deficiency, Lyme, and even cancer. Yet, this is far from a Western or American epidemic. Actually, billions of people all over the world are afflicted.

Most hormonal disorders are never diagnosed. People are ill, and no one knows why. These people may see doctors, but at best they get only a cursory assessment. They may have certain blood tests, including tests for hormone levels, but this is irrelevant. The doctor may notice certain imbalances in the blood work, but rarely is any treatment prescribed. Even so, the measurement of high or low hormone levels is insufficient. This is because the exact hormonal type is never determined. As well, if hormonal disorders are diagnosed, potent and destructive drugs are usually prescribed. Yet, how could this be so? As well, how can drugs be given, which worsen the imbalances? It is because of the fact that doctors are unaware of how to determine the real cause of any imbalance, which is the underlying metabolic type. Regardless, it is the metabolic imbalances, represented by specific body shapes, which are the cause of virtually all diseases.

Despite this, doctors admit that hormonal disorders are relatively common. Specialized blood tests may prove it.

Consider the thyroid gland. Thyroid hormone can be readily measured. This hormone is secreted directly into the blood. In assessing the thyroid a minimum of 20% of individuals demonstrate in their blood evidence of hormonal deficiency. That amounts to a huge number of people. The definition of an epidemic could be easily satisfied if only one percent of the population is sickened. Yet, for instance, up to 60 million Americans suffer from thyroid disorders alone. This means that a huge percentage of the population, up to 40% or more, suffer from hormonal defects.

This is based upon blood tests alone. Astute physicians could confirm this percentage. Is this anything other than the most extreme epidemic conceivable? Yet, if a battery of specialized tests was performed, such as a.m. cortisol, reverse T_3, DHEA, serum estrogen or progesterone, salivary cortisol, serum vitamin D levels, and serum testosterone, an even greater number of cases would be documented. Then, if body types are evaluated, that is to determine the extent of metabolic disorders, along with symptom analysis, the vast majority of Western people would be found to suffer from hormonal imbalance. Thus, rather than an epidemic this is a vast pandemic.

Blood tests only give a hint of the true status. Incredibly, the blood only demonstrates extreme imbalances. Likewise, for it to be demonstrated in the blood it must have existed for a prolonged period, even many years. Yet, through analyzing the body's characteristics and thoroughly reading the features on each individual, the condition may be diagnosed promptly, before the onset of disease. So, in the more subtle cases, where the cause for various symptoms or illnesses is elusive, body typing must be used.

People are sick. Their sicknesses have not been tied to a metabolic factor, even though these people may suspect they have the problem. Often, they complain to the doctor about having a "hormonal imbalance," and in this regard they are usually correct. These cases can be evaluated and discovered, without blood tests. In fact, blood tests may be useless. In contrast, through self-tests and metabolic typing anyone can read his/her body. This book provides the means to do so for each hormonal type. The purpose is to discover the underlying cause for a person's condition. This is so the appropriate treatment can be administered as efficiently as possible and as early as possible. This is to avoid potential disasters. It is so the person can have a better and more productive life. This is through the preventive power of knowing the type and, therefore, administering the ideal treatment. It is also through the power of avoiding based upon this type potentially damaging foods and other substances.

Everyone wishes to feel as good as possible. Yet, for most people it is also important to look as good as possible. Both can be achieved through this book. It is merely necessary to discover the endocrine or metabolic type. As a result, the diet and nutritional program which will best serve each person can finally be determined.

People rely on doctors, but they shouldn't. They should instead rely upon themselves. They should rely upon doctors only for emergencies. Or, the doctor must play the role of diagnostician for preventive purposes. What's more, no one should earn money at the expense of the human body, that is by causing it damage. That would be true fraud.

Yet, no regular doctor knows the endocrine types or how to diagnose them. This book is a guide for people to make their own discoveries. This is the discovery of knowing exactly the metabolic type. Ultimately, people must do all that they can to take responsibility for their own health. They should seek to understand how their bodies work. This will empower them with the knowledge necessary to protect themselves. Such people, armed through education, are, in fact, formidable. This is because they come to know their own bodies instead of relying exclusively on doctors. They will also know their 'metabolic challenges' and how the metabolic/hormone system works. So, they will understand how to correct any imbalances and deficiencies. They also will determine what their bodies need for ideal health. Thus, there is great power in knowing the type.

Such a person is no longer the uneducated, gullible patient. No longer can such a one be swayed to do what could harm the body. Thus, because of this greater awareness to a degree the individual will be protected against medical fraud. When a doctor says something which appears bizarre or which fails to make sense, this person will be hesitant and will seek additional advice. In other words, this person will follow the doctor's advice only if it is truly good for the body. Truly, knowledge is power. It is also protection.

Yet, determining hormonal needs is a challenge. This is because, no doubt, each person is different. The evaluation of thousands of cases has made it clear that people's needs vary greatly. Each person is unique. Truly, again, each person is one-of-a-kind. A single diet for all, for instance, for all overweight people, all heart patients, all diabetics, and all cancer patients, is not acceptable. The diet must be individualized. This can be done through determining the main hormonal types and the two main sub-types. Thus, what is the person's body structure? What is the actual physical appearance? What is the pattern of weight distribution? In other words, what is seen in the mirror? This tells all. Through analyzing this the actual physiology can be determined. Then, this determination is invaluable. What's more, once the body type has been determined treatment can be prescribed accurately.

Not everyone fits the mode perfectly. Thus, there is the occasional variant. However, those who don't fit exactly will at least do so substantially. The challenge is to determine which other component(s) such a person primarily represents. Thus, surely, there are mixed types: there is no "one size fits all." This is why there are sub-types. Yet, the majority of people, some 90%, fit readily into the main four types. This is a system based upon a careful analysis of a person's inborn nature. It is also based upon the obvious exterior features, even bone structure. Of course, the development of the bones is under hormonal control. Thus, the person's type is already established. It only needs to be revealed.

This is a novel approach. As a rule, doctors rely exclusively upon medical tests, as well as a rather brief history and physical, to make the diagnosis. Body types are virtually never considered. Yet, if these were carefully evaluated and the appropriate treatment prescribed, this would revolutionize modern medicine.

Why didn't anyone tell me about this?

No one should expect doctors to know this. Physicians are scientifically trained. They have no interest in analyzing patterns. In contrast, people usually know that their illnesses fit a certain pattern. Yet, people are unable to determine their own health problems. They rightfully expect doctors to discover it. Even so, what they fail to realize is that regarding metabolic or endocrine disorders doctors are woefully ill-informed. Additionally, they have no clue about the role of diet and nutrition in metabolism. Thus, regarding chronic diseases due to impaired metabolism could a doctor's advice be anything except misleading?

Usually, for patients with metabolic disorders most doctors prescribe exclusively drugs. For the symptoms of these disorders, whether physical or mental, additional drugs are prescribed. Drugs interfere with metabolism. They disrupt the endocrine glands. In some cases they even destroy these glands. For instance, the destructive effects of prednisone on the adrenal glands are well known. Regardless, physicians virtually never prescribe natural substances, such as herbs, spice extracts, high-cholesterol foods (as a source of hormonal precursors), root extracts, kelp, vitamins, minerals, and royal jelly, for such disorders. So, in the average doctor's office for any metabolic syndrome dietary and nutritional advice are rarely if ever given.

Incredibly, even if a person has a nutritional deficiency, drugs are the usual treatment. Instead of corrective nutritional therapy the doctor poisons the patient, causing even greater deficiencies. The medical profession gives no credence to the role of diet and nutrition in hormonal disorders. Nor would medical professionals ever admit that roots and herbs are curative and are, in fact, superior to drugs. Yet, nearly always it is the lack of nutrients, as well as hormonal imbalances, which is the cause of metabolic defects.

Rather than drugs in disease the body is deficient in nutrients as well as hormones. The following chart clearly demonstrates this, describing actual physical disorders erroneously treated with drugs:

Metabolic or nutritional disorder	Drug prescribed	Hormonal defect	Nutritional deficiency
depression	antidepressants	thyroid, adrenals	B_6, niacin, thiamine
heartburn	antacids, H-2 blockers	adrenals, thyroid	thiamine, niacin
high cholesterol	statins	thyroid, ovaries, testes	niacin, biotin, essential fatty acids
cancer	chemotherapy	thyroid, adrenals, ovaries	essential fatty acids (EFAs), vitamins C, A, & D
heart disease	calcium-channel blockers, blood thinners, statins	thyroid, adrenals, testes	magnesium, folic acid, B_{12}, selenium, thiamine
diabetes	insulin, hypo-glycemic agents	thyroid, adrenals, liver	thiamine, EFAs niacin, biotin, chromium, magnesium

This chart makes it obvious that diseases are caused by chemical, nutritional, and hormonal imbalances. This is why there is no medical cure for common diseases. This is also why people respond tremendously to the program in this book.

In this metabolic, natural approach both the hormonal and nutrition imbalances are discovered. Then, these conditions are thoroughly treated. This is all done through natural non-toxic means. In medicine neither are treated. Rather, through drug therapy both the metabolic and nutritional processes are corrupted. Drugs destroy hormones. These substances also destroy nutrients. They disable key metabolic agents, particularly enzymes, as well as liver cells. Drugs are horribly toxic to the liver, which is a well-known fact. So, how can they be of any value to the human body?

The body can be fed exactly what it needs based upon its natural tendency. In most people there is a dire lack of the hormones. The body needs these hormones merely to operate, that is to maintain the status quo. This is the endocrine factor that this book emphasizes. It is a factor in everyone's life, especially people living in the Western world.

Why the Western world? Why are people here so vulnerable? It is because of the lifestyle, the diet, and the degree of stress. It is also related to the degree of pollution, which, of course, affects people all over the planet. However, the diet plus stress plays the greatest role. Then, the most damaging diet is the type high in refined carbohydrates and artificial additives. Plus, in the Western diet there is a key imbalance. This is the deficiency of critical substances called hormone precursors. These hormone precursors are systematically stripped from the food. Some 80% of all food consumed in Western countries is heavily processed. In more primitive foods these precursor substances remain intact. Thus, endocrine disorders are truly a Western debacle.

In the fight for survival the endocrine glands are the body's coping mechanism. They alone deal with stress. It's not the brain or the nerves which primarily do so. They are mere end organs, controlled by the glands. Thus, when a person endures stress, when he or she suffers anxiety, depression, feelings of panic, or agitation, when he or she becomes angry or hostile—it is the endocrine glands which must deal with the consequences. Only they can reverse stress-related damage.

These glands are delicate. It takes only minor stresses to upset their chemistry. Dire or uncontrollable stress devastates them. So does a toxic diet. So do nutritional deficiencies. So does exposure to allergens. Additionally, severe psychic strain, frustration, and worry corrupt them. So do even deficiencies of light and healthy air.

In any stress, which obviously includes poor diet, it is, again, the endocrine glands which deal with the consequences. It is they alone which are responsible for reversing the damage. These glands must deal with every conceivable toxicity. Then, the food in the Western world is highly toxic. This is partly due to the high sugar content. Yet, it is also due to the content of poisonous chemicals such as MSG, sulfites, aspartame, sucralose, pesticides, herbicides, and artificial colors/flavors.

The so-called genetically modified foods are another major stressor to the endocrine glands. Genetically modified (GM) means that the food is corrupted by added man-made genes. Such components are known as genetically modified organisms (GMOs). Here, food seeds are developed with artificially altered genes. Yet, rather than being scientific this is all done crudely in a laboratory. The main foods that have been artificially corrupted are corn, soy, cottonseed (used for oil), canola, crooked neck (yellow) squash, and tomatoes. All such genetically altered foods are highly poisonous to the endocrine system.

So, there are many ways a person could be poisoned. For instance, a person eats a sugary pastry or drinks a glass of sugar-infested soda. Or, the person consumes sugar-coated cereal and/or a fake fruit drink. Certainly, such foods/beverages cause hormonal stress. These foods/beverages are infested with refined sugar, refined grains, genetically altered matter, and synthetic chemicals as well as various toxins from mold, pesticides, and herbicides. During metabolism toxic chemicals are produced, such as formaldehyde, acetaldehyde, and methanol, further poisoning the glands. This creates a massive stress on the body. As a result, the body is thrown out of balance. This is where the endocrine glands are critical. These glands systematically strive to correct the imbalances, that is to return the body to normal. This may be difficult, especially if the glands are poisoned.

How could they be poisoned? It is simply as a result of following the typical American diet. Yet, there are other major toxins such as alcohol, caffeine, drugs, food additives, pesticides, herbicides, and various pollutants. Fluoride is yet another highly potent endocrine poison, as are mercury and lead.

Anyone who eats the typical American diet has an endocrine problem. Certainly, such a person's body is functioning below par. Too, the shape readily becomes distorted. Yet, the health can be quickly and dramatically improved. This is through determining the endocrine type and following the specific instructions. In this book each person will find a complete plan for better health. In contrast, there are no cures in modern medicine for endocrine disorders, perhaps with the exception of thyroid hormone for hypothyroidism. Even with this the cure comes at a price: with the synthetic version of this hormone the majority of users develop bone loss, that is osteoporosis. What's more, the drugs that are typically given for other endocrine disorders, for instance, Prednisone or similar steroids for adrenal insufficiency, are so toxic that surely they cause more harm than any benefits. The point is with rare exceptions doctors are unable to help endocrine patients. Often, they cause more harm than good. This demonstrates the importance of determining the metabolic type for supporting the health of each person. The support is achieved through the appropriate diet as well as nutritional supplements and exercise.

There are numerous methods for determining the body or metabolic type. Some of these methods are based upon science. Others are based upon experience, which itself is scientific. This experience reveals that without question each endocrine type is the key to the revival of ideal health. There is no doubt that each person's metabolism is unique. People are physically and structurally different. Anyone can notice this. Just look at a number of people, for instance, walking down the street. Every one of these people is significantly different.

When people go to the doctor, such differences are rarely if ever considered. In fact, these various types are almost never noticed. For instance, if people representing different body/endocrine types were to go to the doctor with, for example, a headache the treatment would be the same. Yet, certainly the treatment must vary based upon the metabolic type. Thus, a headache victim with the thyroid (slow metabolic) type would be given, perhaps, thyroid hormone and iodine-rich food for a headache, as well as herbs, which support the thyroid. Also, the thyroid's sister glands, the ovaries, would be supported nutritionally. In contrast, the adrenal hormonal type would be given pantothenic acid and/or royal jelly, along with certain herbs that support this gland.

The diet would also vary. The adrenal headache victim would be prescribed a moderately high fat/protein diet, along with the elimination of all stimulants. For such a person, cocoa and coffee would be regarded as a poison. A high protein diet, with complex carbohydrates, along with plenty of sea salt, would be prescribed. All food, especially starch and vegetables, would be salted heavily. The point is by normalizing the metabolism through diet and nutritional therapy the headaches can be resolved—without drugs.

This again demonstrates the importance of determining the exact type before prescribing any treatment, including diet. Once the type is determined the precise therapy necessary for ideal health will be known. Now, a person can know the needed diet as well as supplements. This is so that each person can attain the most ideal health possible.

Regarding the issue of a person's physique and even health potential this is to a degree predetermined. Surely, diet also plays a vast role. However, the physiology controls the ultimate result, that is how the shape is formed.

People are concerned about their shape. They are concerned about their appearance. They are also concerned about their actual health. Now, it is possible to control this and cause a rapid improvement. This is by changing the metabolism. The first step is to determine the type. Then, lifelong defects will be corrected. As a result, a person can control both appearance and internal health. When taking corrective measures, the digestion is enhanced. This is a key to ideal physique. There can be a radical change in physique. This enhancement is achieved through metabolic therapy, including diet, herbal medicine, hormonal supplements, exercise, and more.

The Sheldon types

In the Western world there has always been an interest in body types. This led in the early 20th century to a flurry of research. Ultimately, three main types were determined. These types were/are based upon bone structure. The original system was developed by Harvard's Dr. William Sheldon. Based upon extensive research, people are either ectomorphs (*ecto* indicating bones), mesomorphs (*meso* indicating muscle), and endomorphs (*endo* indicating 'internal').

As would be expected the ectomorphs are bony or thin; that is what is noticed the most. In endocrine typing these individuals are usually known as adrenal types. The mesomorphs are noticeably stocky and/or well muscled. Their thick build is highly revealing. They are the typical ball players and/or coaches. They are represented in part by the thyroid-muscular (or muscular-pancreatic) type listed in this book. They may also be thyroid types or thyroid-adrenal types. Endomorphs are noticeably plump or 'abdominal.' They are largely equivalent to the endocrine type known as pituitary or possibly thyroid/adrenal. Regarding the three Harvard types these are definite types, and virtually all people either fit directly into them or a variation thereof.

Sheldon's research is undeniable. It was based upon decades of investigations and hundreds of cases. However, there have been major changes since his time. Today, the issue is far more complex. There is the issue of processed foods, which corrupt the physiology. Now, food is genetically engineered, which accentuates the corruption. Obesity has risen dramatically. Also, people follow various fad diets, which further complicates the issue. Thus, today, body types are not so easily distinguished. True, the three original types still hold true. They form the basis of any body typing attempt: virtually all people still are identifiable by being principally one of Sheldon's types or, perhaps, a combination of them. Yet, today, there is need for an upgrade. The body shape program is that upgrade. It makes sense to classify people. The body is a representation of its function. Peoples' appearances are a real guide. The outer component represents the internal function. What a treasure it is to know and understand the body's needs on an individualized basis. This knowing is a blessing, that each person is individualized by the creator, for those who are desperate for better health. This, then, provides the answers for which people so diligently search, so they can have their health—without medical invasion. For those who have lost all hope, now, there is real hope, because the body reveals all.

For the body typing blood tests tell the bare minimum. The exterior tells far more. So, let's pursue the fascinating journey of learning what your body shape means. As a result, each person's health will dramatically improve. Even the body build and physique will improve. Now, there is hope for all people who suffer from modern diseases. There is also hope for those who desire to feel and look as great as possible for all of their lives. This is through the incredibly valuable system of endocrine/metabolic typing, a system which is revealed by each person's appearance.

Chapter One
Metabolism is the Key

The metabolism is the most critical factor for overall health. Every function in the body is related to it. Every cell and organ in the body is guided by it. What's more, incredibly, through this system the body can be protected from killer diseases.

The metabolism is dependent upon the hormone glands. These glands are known as the endocrine glands. These glands produce powerful hormones, which have major and pervasive actions on the body. Proper weight, strength, beauty, physique, and figure are all under endocrine control. The hormone/endocrine system also controls circulation, digestion, secretion, and elimination. If the metabolism is disordered, the entire body is out of balance. Thus, if the body is working improperly, the first arena to treat is the metabolism. Here, it is necessary to start with a person's nutrition, that is diet. Also, the appropriate supplements must be prescribed to correct the metabolic defects.

The body types—the endocrine types—have a direct relation to a person's diet. This is through human physiology. Physiology is how the body works. Each person's body operates in a unique fashion. So, the actual metabolism in each person is different. When a person needs dietary or nutritional support or when he or she needs guidance in the treatment of disease, these rules, that is the function of specific body types, must be taken into account. Put simply, to best help a person the exact nature of how the body works must be known. This may be regarded as "individualized physiology."

Everyone is different. This is easily realized. Just take time to look at a number of people, for instance, people walking down a busy street or in a mall. All such people are unique. This is an astounding element, a kind of proof of the creative powers.

This is supported by divine revelation. In the magnificent holy books the almighty creator makes it clear that every person is a created being. He also makes it clear that each person is unique, a fact, for instance, found in the Qur'aan. Here, the individuality of each person is described, down to "the fingertips." This wisdom is found universally. If people are different in appearance, then, surely, they are also different functionally. Surely, even their precise organs and genes are different. Thus people are individuals, and regarding health individual differences must be considered. This can easily be achieved through the metabolic typing system. In fact, such typing is the secret to gaining profound health. It is also the secret to determining which foods a person should or shouldn't eat.

The hormonal glands are responsible for metabolism. The body shape plus various symptoms reveals the health or lack thereof of those glands. It is the metabolism which determines virtually all aspects of health: a person's vitality, mental status, physical strength, immune status, and physique. Other factors besides the metabolism will be considered. Yet, these factors operate to a large degree by influencing the metabolism.

People are confused about what they should eat. Once the nature of the metabolism is discovered, then, the person can follow the right diet. All the plans, low-carbohydrate, vegetarianism, veganism, macrobiotic, and raw food, are irrelevant until this is uncovered.

Truly, people are confused. This is because they receive a litany of messages. Try this or that diet, they are told. Eat meat or avoid meat. White meat is better than red. Red meat causes cancer. Eat eggs or avoid eggs. Eat only raw foods. Consume lots of whole grains or restrict grains. Eat mostly complex carbohydrates or restrict carbohydrates. Eat fruit for breakfast or eat mostly protein. These are all generalities, which may hold some truth but which, certainly, cause great confusion. What is lacking is a system for determining a person's exact needs based upon the actual type of body and physiology rather than vague generalities.

The factors which must be considered in individualizing the diet include genetic origin, which is dealt with through the blood type, race, climate, that is where the person currently lives, the personal physiological type, and, of course, the endocrine or metabolic type. The latter tells of the nature of a person's physiology more so than any other factor, including the blood. Other factors include previous medical history, nutritional status, food allergies, immune health, and any history of exposure to toxins or germs. Serious medical illnesses also play a significant role in determining the body's needs.

A serious medical illness can, in fact, alter the body type, eventually shifting a person from one body type to another. Surgery may particularly do so, especially if key hormonal organs, such as the thyroid or ovaries, are damaged or destroyed. Also, where a person lives has a significant impact, particularly if the area is heavily polluted or if it is in the extreme of climates.

The role of climate is significant. There are certain foods and nutrients which must be consumed to protect against cold weather. Virtually all such nutrients are found in animal foods. Thus, a vegetarian diet is catastrophic in northern climates, especially in people of northern European stock. Must a person, therefore, follow such a diet, merely because one factor, such as blood, deems it? This has no scientific basis. The ideal diet depends upon a variety of factors, although the hormone/metabolic type is, perhaps, most critical.

This metabolic imprint is revealed by each person's body. It is made obvious by a person's body structure, that is physique, and especially the face as well as head. It is revealed by the bone structure, the behavior, and even the walk. The metabolic type supercedes the climate, the blood, or any other factor.

Regardless of where a person lives or his genetics it will reveal what is the primary diet, which can be modified based upon other significant factors, including genetics, climate, region, and heritage. Thus, a northern Russian, Canadian, or European who is a pituitary type has many of the same dietary and nutritional needs of, for instance, an Egyptian or African with the same type. However, like his northern counterpart the Egyptian or African would ideally modify his diet based upon climate.

Carbohydrates, easily metabolized in hot climates, would ideally represent a considerable portion of the diet, for instance, local fruit, although protein would also be necessary. Instead of the typical advice for the pituitary type—the addition of large amounts of fatty fish—the subtropical person would ideally eat non-fatty fish and lots of it, which is more readily metabolized in the hot Mediterranean climate than the fatty carbohydrates. Regardless of the body type fresh seafood from the region would also be on the platter. What's more, fatty fish would be difficult to find in Egypt or Central Africa, whereas the higher protein whitefish are commonly found.

Fatty fish oils are insulators. In other words, they cause the retention of heat. In hot climates in particular there is no need to consume large quantities of such fish/fish oils. Again, the fats in these fish or fish oil supplements cause heat retention, which is the opposite of what is desired. Nor would a diet of fatty beef be advisable. Nor in the tropics or subtropics would the regular consumption of large amounts of butterfat or cream be advisable. This is because in a hot climate the consumption of fat, as well as protein, causes heat retention, while the consumption of carbohydrate dissipates heat. Such heat retention is of value in cold climates, therefore, the fat- and protein-rich diet of the Inuit and/or northern Siberian.

Fatty foods are rich sources of vitamins A and D. Yet, the intake of such foods is far more necessary in cold climates than in the hot tropics or sub-tropics. In particular, regarding the latter sunlight provides for vitamin D synthesis.

The endocrine glands: key to body typing

Within the body there are twelve critical endocrine glands. Each of these glands is necessary for survival. Each controls vital functions. Each secretes incredibly potent substances, which are absolutely vital. These vital substances are known as secretory factors. These secretory factors, of which there are dozens, ultimately are converted into endocrine hormones. An imbalance or deficiency in any one of these hormones may rapidly precipitate symptoms and disease, even death.

Secretory function is largely dependent upon sunlight. It is the sunlight which activates the key glands, the pituitary and the pineal, which control endocrine function. With no sunlight, the endocrine secretions quickly become depleted and the glands dysfunctional. Sunlight itself is a cure for endocrine disorders.

The secretions of the endocrine glands are essential to health. The glands which activate the endocrine system, the pineal and pituitary, are found in the brain. So is the hypothalmus, which is the ultimate control center for hormones. Here, the hormone glands and organs are centrally placed. Yet, so are the glands in the rest of the body such as the thyroid and parathyroid glands, the thymus, the adrenals, one on each side of the spine, the stomach, and the gonads.

Even so, no one knows for certain exactly what the endocrine glands do. This fact supports a more naturalistic approach to treatment. Medical research has determined a portion of their functions. Certainly, it is known that they each secrete hormones. It is also known that such hormones target certain organs. Some of these hormones have been synthesized. For these synthetic hormones a certain mechanism of action is known. Yet, the majority of their actions remain unknown. Plus, there are, certainly, within the body a variety of hormones yet to be discovered. All that is truly known is that endocrine glands secrete fluids containing powerful compounds. These compounds have specific effects upon cells and organs throughout the body. Thus, the secretions of the endocrine glands control how the body operates: the whole body. When an endocrine gland unleashes its secretions, the blood and lymph carry it to all parts of the body, in fact, every cell. This is true of all endocrine glands. This means that if such a secretion is deficient, all cells are adversely affected. Thus, it is no surprise that systemic diseases, such as obesity, heart disease, arthritis, mental diseases, lupus, diabetes and cancer, are directly correlated to disturbed endocrine function.

The point is the endocrine glands secrete a transparent fluid into the blood and lymph, which is complex in nature. There is no way to know for certain the exact chemistry of this fluid. Some of the chemistry is known, for instance, that the secretion from the thyroid gland contains thyroxine. Thus, chemists have made a synthetic version. However, there must be other components of the secretion, which are unknown. This explains the failure to cure with synthetic preparations.

There is no way to support the metabolic type with such formulations. For instance, when synthetic thyroxine is taken in "physiological doses" over prolonged periods it usually causes side effects, including bone loss and heart rhythm disturbances. In contrast, the naturally produced thyroid secretion, which is a complexity of multiple substances, never causes these negative effects. Rather, the natural complexes, for instance, the combination of crude types of kelp from the far northern oceans, with the amino acid tyrosine and wild oregano, actually increases bone density. The same is true of other preparations, such as truly organic glandulars, liquid or dry extract of maca root, and royal jelly. The latter crude and low dose substances actually help normalize metabolic function. Great improvement is achieved through the intake of such a whole food formula. This proves that endocrine secretions are more complicated than is known. There is another important point, which explains the nature of this system. The body never works in isolation. There are never separate glands that work independently. All 12 or so endocrine glands work as a team, like a symphony of an orchestra. If one player is out of balance, it affects the entire unit, and this imbalance is always noticeable, usually through predictable symptoms. It may even be manifested by certain diseases, some of which can be lethal. Yet, all these symptoms and diseases can be reversed by, first, discovering the metabolic type and, then, applying appropriate treatment, without drugs or surgery.

As reported by the endocrine gland surgeon Dr. T. H. Larson it was known as early as the 1920s that the endocrine glands operate essentially as a "single unit." Let this be absolutely clear: a relatively minor disturbance in a gland can dramatically upset the entire system. The key is balance. Here, the individual achieves help achieving this balance in a natural and safe way.

Because of the modern way of living this balance has been disrupted. Poor diet and, thus, nutritional deficiency plays a major role in disturbing this function. So does stress. These glands are immediately disrupted by psychic pressures. Any emotional distress or negativity direly affects them. In particular, worry greatly disrupts them. Trust and confidence have the opposite effect. In fact, positive emotions, the emotions of love, and peace—keep them in balance.

While in general the system is symphonic there are certain specific actions that the endocrine glands exert upon specific regions. In fact, one organ may largely control another. For instance, the adrenal glands dramatically affect the sex glands, while the parathyroid gland dramatically influences the bones and joints. In females, the ovaries exert major actions upon the breasts and thyroid. Thus, the glands and organs are intertwined. One cannot suffer from an imbalance in a specific gland without the whole system being affected. If the action of one is reduced, there is a definite negative action on the related organ or gland. Thus, as a general rule, if the ovaries are diseased, the thyroid is also diseased. If there is disease in the parathyroid glands, the bones, as well as thyroid, are also diseased. If the ovaries are corrupted, so will be the adrenals and vice versa. If the testes are disturbed, so will be the adrenals and vice versa. The connection is direct. So is the influence.

If the digestion is adequate, there is good health. The physique and the body shape are balanced. Failure to properly digest food results in poor health. Yet, the entire digestive process is controlled by the hormones. So, poor digestion and distorted physique are ultimately due to hormonal factors.

Proof for the existence of metabolic defects is glaring. Surely, this is monumentally true in Western countries. It has already been stated that impairment of metabolism results in distortion of the physique. For instance, in the United States six of ten Americans are overweight. These Americans constantly struggle to lose weight. For most overweight people dieting alone is largely inadequate. Solving the metabolic crisis is far more effective, because defects of metabolism are the basis of the weight gain. This weight is held within the body to absorb the toxicity of vast cellular imbalances. The imbalances are caused by metabolic defects, which, can be due to deficiencies as well as toxicities. The ingestion of poisonous foods and chemicals may play a greater role in obesity than even caloric intake. Such toxic foods/chemicals disable the function of the endocrine glands, which may result in weight gain. This weight may be represented both by actual fat as well as fluid retention. This is why dieting alone rarely solves the disorder.

For obese people solving the metabolic disorder can lead to rapid and effective weight loss. What's more, unlike dieting, this is a regimen which can be followed for a prolonged period. Regardless, any diet must be easy to follow. The food must also be tasty and sufficiently filling that a person continues to follow it, perhaps indefinitely. Plus, it must be somewhat flexible. In this fast-paced world there is little time for food preparation. The diet must be adaptable to all people regardless of circumstances. Thus, relying on complex recipes isn't always feasible. Even so, people must make up their minds to prepare their own food—if they wish to achieve the greatest benefits from this program. Yet, it is more than for mere weight loss. This is a lifestyle program for all people who desire ideal health.

Who has time to cook? To lose weight, usually, there is need to prepare food. To become more beautiful it is necessary to make an effort: to prepare healthy food. However, on this diet there are both simple meals and also complex ones. There are meals which take only a few minutes and others which take, perhaps, hours. If time is an issue, use the simpler recipes and modify other recipes for this purpose. Since some of the advice is exotic, rather, cumbersome it may be regarded as 'optional.'

There is no need to follow everything exactly. If there are items which are difficult to find or foods which are unavailable, work around this. Follow the main concepts.

In this diet there are no processed foods. This is particularly true of the so-called genetically engineered foods. These foods should be avoided at all costs. They cause significant health damage, plus they are a major cause of allergic reactions. Strict avoidance of such foods is necessary, because such foods are a major cause of illness, including obesity. With these foods there is a high tendency for allergic reactions. Yet, these reactions may not be acute, in other words, they may be subtle and chronic. Rather, than obvious allergic symptoms, such as hives, rashes, itching, runny nose, and fits of sneezing, these reactions are usually manifested by chronic problems such as digestive disturbances, bloating, sinus problems, weakened immune system, swelling, skin rashes, breathing disorders, and, of course, weight gain. The main foods which are genetically engineered include commercial corn and corn products, and soy derivatives, canola, and cottonseed.

Food additives must also be strictly avoided. They also disrupt body chemistry, causing a wide range of symptoms. Weight loss can result simply by avoiding such additives. Many of these additives cause significant tissue damage, even causing serious diseases such as attention deficit disorder, autism, asthma, and cancer. The majority of food additives are synthetic chemicals, made, incredibly, from petrol or coal tar. The majority of these chemicals are proven carcinogens and, thus, are unfit for human consumption. Thus, it is no surprise that their ingestion leads to a wide range of physiological imbalances, weight gain, swelling, and bloating being merely a few of the manifestations. The point is if a person wishes to lose weight and keep it off, it is necessary to strictly avoid all foods containing toxic additives.

To discover the metabolic type is a tool to create balance in these glands. It is also a tool to prevent the onset of significant disease, both of the endocrine system and elsewhere. The metabolic type is the window to future success. The energy level, the physical desires, the emotions, the mental capacity, and even the career are dependent upon it. Again, this is based upon the actual physical structure of the body.

The primary metabolic types include the pituitary type, which is the rarest, the adrenal type, the thyroid type, and the thyroid-adrenal type. These are known as the four common endocrine types. There are other types, so that the total types may truly number a dozen or more. However, virtually all people fit primarily into one of the four main types and the two sub- or combination types.

People are basically born with their types. These inherent types can become modified over time as a result of certain influences, including poor diet and stress. Even so, the main type is fixed. A person can never escape his or her type. Thus, for any individual the metabolic type acts as a guide in order to read the individual's physical and personal needs as well as design the appropriate diet.

Everyone fits a specific pattern. Some of these patterns are easy to determine, because they are pure types, fitting the metabolic profile clearly. Others are more difficult; they are the combined types. The issue is to determine a person's type to maximize his or her health. Once identified, an accurate diet can be designed, which is based upon each person's specific physiology.

Metabolism as a system

There is a science to estimating metabolism. This science is based upon the body's surface area. This is because experiments have shown that the inherent metabolic rate has more to do with the surface area of a person's body than just the weight. This means that the bone structure, height, and weight must all be considered. For instance, consider two men of the same weight, though one is much taller than the other. Because of his height the taller one has more surface area. As a result, his metabolism is higher, perhaps 10% or more.

This may cause a degree of confusion. What about a very heavy man? He will also have a larger surface area than a thin man, for instance, of the same height. Even so, it has been determined that the thinner man, despite a slightly less surface area, has a faster metabolic rate, which, obviously, explains why he is thin. Incredibly, the difference in metabolic rate between the broader man and his thinner counterpart can be as much as 35%, that is the burning of 35% more food every day than the obese person. Thus, if two men of approximately the same weight are measured, it is the taller one who usually has the higher metabolic activity.

Even two people who appear the same and who have the same height and weight may dramatically differ in their metabolism. One explanation is that the major arena of metabolism is the muscles. The size of the muscles in individuals may differ without necessarily causing a difference in weight. For instance, a person can have big bones but relatively small muscles. Such a person would have a lower metabolic rate than a person with a medium frame and larger muscles. A woman and man may weigh the same, but women usually have a higher density of fat tissue in relation to muscle than men. Thus, the woman has a lower metabolic rate. Plus, because she naturally has a higher number of fat cells, she is highly vulnerable to the deposition of fat. If both eat the same amount of food, it is the woman who will invariably gain weight. This is why it is so crucial to determine the body type, so that the metabolic pattern can be appropriately treated. By adjusting the diet to meet the metabolic needs weight challenges are both reversed and prevented.

Certain factors directly alter metabolism. These factors include mental status, that is mental stress, exercise, age, and weather. Cold weather generally increases metabolism, while hot weather can in some individuals slow it. Incredibly, a cold shower can dramatically increase metabolism, doubling oxygen consumption. A person exposed to a blustery cold climate, like an Alpine mountain resident or an Inuit, might endure a 40% to 70% increase in metabolic rate. This demonstrates the crucial nature of climate and food. Obviously, in cold climate the need for efficient fuel is great. This will be discussed in more detail later.

With age metabolism declines. At age forty significant decreases are noticed, which means that after forty people are unable to burn food as aggressively. It is well known that at this age changes in body conformation occur, and the weight gain seems to happen suddenly. This is due to changes in how fast the body burns fuel. Thus, after forty the body's need for calories significantly declines. At 60 the decline is substantial. People should consider reducing their total food consumption as they age, since that is the natural tendency.

It is well known that disorders of the endocrine glands greatly alter metabolism. These disorders also disrupt digestion. As a result, how the body processes food is greatly impacted. Disorders of the thyroid gland are excellent examples. Excessive thyroid secretion, that is hyperthyroidism, may increase the metabolic rate some 75%. This leads to the excessive burning of fuel and, usually, a thin or emaciated condition. As well, sluggish thyroid secretion, that is hypothyroidism, may decrease it by as much as 30%. This results in fatigue, impaired or 'slow' digestion, and also weight gain. Insufficient pituitary secretions may reduce the metabolism an additional 5%. As a result, usually, the individual becomes bloated, swollen, and readily gains weight. Again, this weight gain may either be represented as blocked/retained fluids or fat deposition or a combination thereof. Sluggish adrenal gland function may result in a 5% to 10% decline in metabolic rate.

The endocrine secretions are tremendously powerful. Dumped into the blood, as well as lymph, the components of these secretions react within the cells immediately. According to Herman Pomerantz in his book *The Family Physician* endocrine secretions are the body's natural drugs. This is an incredible but true comparison. The endocrine hormones are the most potent substances known and are in many instances hundreds of times more potent than any known drug. If a gland is named as part of the endocrine system, this means a simple fact: it is a hormone-producing factory. Fritz Kahn, M.D., calls these hormones "chemical messengers."

It may only take an infinitesimal amount of such chemical messengers to achieve the desired result. The body needs such rapid action. The endocrine glands are the fast reactors, which protect the human being against every conceivable danger. Once these hormones enter the bloodstream, their actions are immediate and systemic. No cell escapes their potent influence. In fact, they are the most potent and effective of all substances produced by the human body.

Chapter Two

The Endocrine System: An Overview

There are eight main endocrine glands. These glands are the pituitary, pineal, thyroid, thymus parathyroid, adrenals, pancreas, ovaries, and testes. There are four ancillary glands which produce hormones or hormone-like substances. These are the stomach, liver, kidneys, and skin. So, essentially, there are twelve endocrine systems.

Pituitary

Located at the base of the brain, this is regarded as the true master of the endocrine system. In fact, it exerts a degree of control over each of the main glands. It is located next to the junction of the optic nerves. The optic nerve arises in the eyes. It sends signals from the eyes to the brain. These signals are obviously absorbed by the pituitary, which rests atop this nerve. This demonstrates the importance of daylight in the gland's function. Sunlight activates this organ. Darkness calms or de-activates it. The eyes activate the secretion of "controlling hormones." These are hormones which modify and instruct the function of the other key endocrine glands: the thyroid, adrenals, pancreas, liver, ovaries, and testes. The breasts are also under its influence. Thus, milk production is largely controlled by the pituitary. The list of organs or body regions influenced by this gland includes the thyroid, bones, pancreas, adrenal glands, testes, ovaries, uterus, mammary glands, arteries, skin, nervous system, intestinal tract, skeleton, muscular system, heart, and kidneys. Thus, it exerts influence over all major organ systems.

Growth of the human body is largely controlled by the pituitary. This is because it produces a potent substance known as growth hormone. The great changes in youngsters during puberty are a consequence of its actions. In particular, pituitary hormone acts upon the skeleton, dramatically changing it. This is largely through the actions of growth hormone. Thus, if there is a failure to grow in youngsters, usually this is due to pituitary malfunction, although thyroid disorders also often play a role. This gland also directly influences the muscles, increasing muscular strength as well as growth. Thus, it is obvious that this gland influences the structure and even formation of the body.

Fat deposition is also under pituitary control. So is its metabolism. In disease of this gland the metabolism of fat is greatly decreased. Thus, fat deposits readily form. This is largely because of disabled carbohydrate metabolism, that is where the starch and sugar which is consumed is poorly or incompletely burned. Thus, it is converted in the liver to fat and, then, deposited throughout the body.

Pineal

Like the pituitary, this gland is found within the brain substance. It is activated by light and influences sleep. What is little known is that the pineal gland plays a great role in sexual development. It directly promotes sexual maturity. This gland also influences the proper maturation of the adolescent mind. A disturbance in it could lead to a retardation of mental development.

This may explain the toxic effects of computers, as well as cell phones, on brain cells, especially in youth. This is because the pineal gland is highly sensitive to light and radiation-related stimuli. The high amount of radiation, plus the artificial light, plus the intense stimulation from computer games and cell phones, greatly upsets the chemistry of this gland. This can result in a wide range of mental symptoms including insomnia, mental instability, irritability, visual disorders, fatigue, and even violent propensities.

The pineal gland secretes a critical compound known as melatonin. This substance is involved in the maintenance of proper sleep. It also helps balance the immune system. Its powers regarding the immune system are vast. In fact, melatonin is one of the body's main systems for preventing the development of cancer. It also keeps the immune cells in ideal activity to prevent various infections. Plus, it directly impacts aging, exerting a general action to prevent the breakdown of the body. In this regard it is a potent antioxidant, which has a positive action on all cells throughout the body.

Ultimately, the pineal as well as the pituitary are under the control of the brain. It is this organ which controls the hormone system. This is through the secretion of special hormones, known as hypothalamic releasing factors, which act on these glands. The pineal gland is also regarded as the spiritual center of the body, which may explain how light or a lack thereof really influences it.

Thyroid

This gland is known as the master of metabolism. The thyroid gland produces three main hormones. The key ones, thyroxine and triiodothyronine, control the metabolic rate. What is metabolism? *Dorland's Medical Dictionary* defines it as two life-giving processes. First, there is anabolism, which is "the sum of all the physical and chemical processes by which living organized substance is produced and maintained." Then, there is catabolism, which is "the transformation by which energy is made available for the uses of the organism." Furthermore, basal metabolism, which the thyroid largely controls, is defined as "the minimal energy expended for the maintenance of respiration, circulation, peristalsis (that is the normal movements of the gut), muscle tone, body temperature, glandular activity, and other... functions of the body."

The thyroid gland is extensively involved in growth and development. In other words, for a person to develop from a baby onward, in fact, in the womb it is necessary for this gland to function optimally. Consider its role in bone tissue. According to Le Gros-Clark in *Tissues of the Body* for bones to lengthen thyroid hormone is essential. He describes the results of experiments where the thyroid was removed from young animals. This results in a vast inhibition of bone growth. Thus, the person with stunted growth likely suffers from a thyroid defect.

Also, the sex glands are under thyroid control. In particular, for females the function of all female glands is greatly influenced by this organ. Thus, any disorder of the female reproductive system may be due to a thyroid imbalance.

How can a single gland accomplish all this? It is through its mechanism of action. Thyroid hormones regulate the metabolic rate by acting directly upon the cells. They do this through stimulating cellular enzymes. Thus, thyroid hormone excites the enzymes into action. The thyroid gland also produces thyrocalcitonin. As the name implies this hormone causes calcium to be deposited into bone. It also acts on the kidneys, causing them to decrease their excretion of this mineral. Therefore, thyrocalcitonin is crucial for maintaining skeletal health.

Thus, there are numerous hormones produced by this gland. This is also why whole food supplements, such as crude remote-source bull kelp concentrates and organic whole food glandulars, balance the thyroid gland better than isolates.

Thyroid hormone is secreted into the blood in an inactive form. It is activated in the liver through enzymatic reaction. Thus, healthy liver function is essential for adequate thyroid function.

Parathyroid

The prefix para means "besides." The parathyroid glands are located on the backside of the thyroid lobes, two on each side. Larson claims this gland is involved with the deposition of fat. Modern textbooks give it only one job: the metabolism of calcium and phosphorus.

These glands, although tiny, are utterly critical. Their removal results in death, usually within a few days. This demonstrates the critical importance of calcium in the body, as well as phosphorus, both of which are controlled by these glands. The parathyroid hormones act mainly upon three organ systems: the digestive system, the kidneys, and the bones. Along with vitamin D, parathyroid hormones accelerate calcium absorption. With this organ two types of syndromes occur. These are sluggish function, known as hypoparathyroidism, and excessive function, known as hyperparathyroidism. These syndromes appear to be equally common. In both cases the consequences are due to disturbed calcium and phosphorus balance. A low blood calcium level is a sign of hypoparathyroidism, while a high level signals hyperparathyroidism.

Pancreas

The pancreas produces a wide range of substances. It is included in the endocrine system mainly because of one of these substances, which is insulin. This hormone is produced by a group of cells, known as beta cells, located in the far end, that is the tail. It is involved chiefly with carbohydrate metabolism. This appears to be the main purpose of the pancreas, since the beta cells constitute about 75% of its weight.

Insulin is a potent hormone. It aggressively acts upon the body's main fuel molecule, glucose, driving it into cells. The main site of this action is the muscles. However, it also acts upon the fat cells. This is an unhealthy consequence, since these cells deposit the glucose as fat.

According to Tuttle's *Textbook of Physiology* there is normally a barrier to the entry of glucose into the cells. It is insulin which overcomes this barrier, forcing the entry of this molecule into the cell matrix. Exercise is another factor precipitating glucose entry, since this burns existing energy stores, causing cells to open up their glucose barriers. The pancreas also produces glucagon. This is insulin's opposite. The body produces it in response to blood sugar levels, which are too low. Thus, it helps the body raise blood sugar levels.

An excess of insulin is highly dangerous. This leads to the so-called syndrome X. This syndrome is associated with a high risk for heart disease and diabetes. In syndrome X, as well as diabetes, the insulin levels are not necessarily high. Low insulin levels are associated with Type I diabetes. Thus, the key to ideal hormonal health is to maintain stable blood sugar levels. This would surely help prevent the onset of diabetes as well as its precursor syndrome X. This is through causing insulin to be used more readily. Here, the intake of potent spice extracts, such as a multiple spice oil concentrate, including oils of cumin, wild oregano, wild myrtle, and cinnamon, is ideal. In health food stores look for the multiple spice extract which has been demonstrated to greatly aid insulin function. It is a key formula for reversing the metabolic defects in syndrome X and similar disorders related to disordered blood sugar metabolism. It is even effective against diabetes.

Another ideal remedy is CO_2 extracted cinnamon bark. Ideally, this can be taken as drops from a one-ounce bottle under the tongue. It must not be a tincture but rather the oil in extra virgin olive oil, again, cold-extracted. This extraction method causes the retention of the antihyperglycemic flavonoids in an unaltered form. Again, look for CO_2 extracted cinnamon bark as drops in extra virgin olive oil. This is a tasty way to reverse syndrome X and fight carbohydrate intolerance. Because of the taste, it is ideal for children and teenagers.

Ovaries

These are the key glands for maintaining femininity. They play an enormous role in the vital womanhood that all women desire. They are what give a woman her beauty and fertility. If they are functioning properly, a woman looks like a woman, with the proper body curves and skin tone. If their function is compromised, the female characteristics can be disrupted or lost.

In fact, in the complete ovarian failure women can lose their natural beauty. They may become too thin or heavy. The formation about their hips and waists becomes distorted. They can even develop male characteristics, including a masculine-like bone structure and hair in a male-pattern. The ovaries control a woman's appearance as well as spirit. Thus, a vivacious woman is one who has healthy ovaries. Mentally and physically for a woman to be healthy the ovaries must be healthy.

The ovaries are the source of a wide range of feminizing hormones. If produced in sufficient quantities, these hormones may improve a woman's physical features. Through a natural endocrine therapy aimed at these organs the women's bodies could be completely revitalized. The degree of this organ's feminizing power is illustrated by early research. As reported by Steinbach in *Organotherapy* if the ovaries are transplanted into a castrated male, his body converts to a female type. The male even develops functional breasts.

The power of the ovaries is demonstrated by a simple fact. It begins with a girl's body. That body is not truly female. How, then, does such an immature body become transformed into the body of a woman? It is the ovaries which are responsible for this transformation. Womanhood is far from merely an accident. The ovaries make it deliberate. If these organs are destroyed, essentially, womanhood is lost.

It is these glands which are responsible for a woman's shapely figure as well as any libido. Regarding the latter, it is well known that if a woman loses her ovaries, her libido often collapses. What's more, experiments have shown that if a teenager develops ovarian disease or if her ovaries are removed, this greatly disturbs body conformation. Obesity usually results, and, certainly, the woman's life is made miserable. Health declines and is often manifested as the onset of serious diseases, including heart disease, cancer, high blood pressure, and diabetes.

The activity of the ovaries is far from a miracle. It is due to specific chemical substances, which nourish and activate these glands. The main agents responsible are the lipids, that is cholesterol-like molecules. That cholesterol is largely responsible for ovarian powers can be confirmed by any anatomist or surgeon: the ovaries are so full of this substance that they have a waxy appearance, being tinged yellow by it. This has also been confirmed by numerous researchers, who have determined that if these fats, more correctly, lipids are extracted and given medicinally, they produce all the results expected of the ovaries. Therefore, in the human body lipids, particularly cholesterol, play a life-supporting role.

The chemistry of the ovaries is easily disturbed. In this regard there are two distinct syndromes. These are sluggish function and excessive function. Symptoms of sluggish function include low body temperature, small or malformed breasts, immature sex gland development, small uterus, scanty or irregular menses, and obesity. Regarding this constellation of disorders this often signifies the plump and often infertile female. Typically, a person with sluggish ovaries has a predictable body type: either tall and lanky or obese. Often, such persons deposit much weight on their outer hips, especially below the hip socket. With excessive function there is rapid sexual maturity at too young an age, early onset of teeth formation, early menstruation, early appearance of pubic and armpit hair, and premature development of sexual function and desire. The youngster with excessive function is often the one who has an excessively strong sex desire at too young an age. This symptom may actually be correctable through nutritional therapy.

The ovaries are part of a complete system of hormone glands. Dysfunction in these organs can disrupt the entire hormone system. In particular, healthy ovarian function is dependent upon normal functioning of the thyroid gland, adrenal glands, and pituitary gland. A high intake of sugar is particularly disruptive to these glands, as is an excessively low-fat diet. In particular, pregnant and nursing women should never follow a either a low-fat or high-sugar diet, as this causes ovarian failure.

Testes

The main purpose of these glands is the manufacture of the male sex hormone testosterone. This hormone, while involved in sperm production, is a major factor in a man's strength. It largely controls the creation of muscle tissue. It also creates physical and mental power. It is the primary source of a man's sexual strength. During early development testosterone helps facilitate bone development. It aids in amino acid metabolism by increasing the utilization of these nutrients within the liver and kidneys. What's more, this hormone has a general tonic effect upon the body, increasing, as it does in puberty, the overall metabolism. If secreted in significant amounts, it creates a "sense of well being." Zoth and Pregl found early in the 1900s that when extra testosterone was injected in men combined with an aggressive exercise program muscular strength increased some 50%. The active ingredients of the testes are, like those of the ovaries, derivatives of cholesterol. Therefore, a low cholesterol diet can cause atrophy of these glands as well as muscle collapse. This atrophy and/or muscle damage can also be a consequence of taking cholesterol-lowering drugs. Men on low cholesterol diets are usually feeble. To gain their male strength they must eat cholesterol-rich foods and/or foods with testosterone precursors. Natural, organic sources of testosterone or its precursors include organ meats, fatty fish, organic fresh red meat, royal jelly, crude cold-pressed sesame oil, tahini, crude cold-pressed pumpkinseed oil, cold-extracted purple maca root extract, wild sarsaparilla berry extract, and pumpkin seeds.

Adrenal glands

These glands are the key system for dealing with stress. They produce cortisone and adrenalin, two of the body's key anti-stress hormones.

The adrenal glands are essential for survival. If they are removed, death occurs precipitously. Damage to the adrenal glands, especially the central part of the cortex, leads to great health problems. In the extreme this is known as Addison's disease. This disease is so serious that it is regarded as fatal. Yet, there are many levels of lesser damage, not enough to kill but enough to cause major disruption. This is known as *subclinical Addison's syndrome*. It is exceedingly common in people who follow a Western diet.

These glands are directly involved with the growth of the organs as well as the skeleton. They also play a major role in sexual development. The precise maintenance of life, of a person's actual existence, is dependent upon them. The adrenal glands also affect body conformation, for instance, the structure of the muscles and the bones as well as the dentition. A person with feeble adrenal production is, in fact, weak, while in contrast a person with adequate or high production is strong. A person with greatly impaired adrenal function is often physically feeble to such a degree that routine tasks are impossible. In contrast, a person with powerful production is strong with a robust physique and plenty of energy. However, in modern civilization the latter is rare.

The adrenal glands control a vast number of functions. These include the maintenance of the levels of body fluids, salt and water metabolism, heart pumping power, blood pressure, fertility, libido, digestion, the combating of toxicity, blood sugar regulation, and muscular strength as well as stamina. A person with strong adrenal glands is the ideal athlete. A person with weak glands is better served as an intellectual. In fact, the typical intellectual or, today, the 'computer geek' is usually the adrenal type.

These glands make key hormones needed to fight infection as well as inflammation. Adrenal hormones are also needed to protect the body against allergic reactions. They also make a critical hormone associated with longevity. This is DHEA (dihydroxyepiandosterone), which is a measure of life span. Low levels of DHEA is a sign of the potential for premature death.

The stress response depletes these glands. This is true to a degree of physical stress. However, these organs are even more greatly disrupted by psychic stress. Thus, any type of mental aberration, such as worry, frustration, grief, depression, and anxiety, leads to dysfunction. For the adrenals the worst emotion is anger. This devastates their function.

The adrenals are aided by fatty foods, especially those rich in cholesterol. The latter is the raw material for the production of the vast majority of adrenal hormones. Foods rich in cholesterol include fatty fish, seafood, fish eggs, fatty salmon oil (steam extracted, polar source), red meat, organ meats, poultry (with the skin on), whole milk, butter, yogurt, quark, and kefir. Salt also aids adrenal function by causing the conservation of the hormone aldosterone. Unprocessed complex carbohydrates may be well tolerated, especially when eaten with plenty of fat and salt. In contrast, the adrenal glands are readily damaged by refined carbohydrates, especially white sugar and corn syrup.

Thymus

Located behind the upper part of the breast bone the thymus is primarily an immune gland. The main job of this gland is to produce hormones, which activate the immune system. These thymic hormones cause the body to produce white blood cells. The thymus acts largely upon the bone marrow and lymph glands, where it activates cell synthesis. Thymic hormones act like antibiotics, aiding in the destruction of invasive germs. Zinc is needed for thymic hormone activity. A severe deficiency of this mineral can essentially halt the function of this gland.

The thymus gland is highly vulnerable to toxins. In particular, vaccines intoxicate it. Repeated vaccinations result in the destruction of this gland. As a result, it is difficult to activate. This is why vaccines readily lead to immune deficiency and even cancer.

Radiation also destroys this gland. Anyone who has had repeated X-rays, radiation therapy, and/or CAT scans is likely to have severe thymic damage. Radiation causes fungal overgrowth. It also destroys the bone marrow as well as the lymph nodules. Then, the immune system of anyone undergoing radiation therapy is generally under siege. Here, it is necessary to boost the function of the thymus gland with natural medicines.

Natural spice oils help activate the thymus gland. These spice oils, for instance, oil of wild oregano, wild sage oil, and wild lavender oil, can be rubbed on the upper sternum, which is the thymic reflex. This can be done ideally at night before bedtime. The most powerful of these is wild oregano oil in the form of Mediterranean-source wild hand-picked oregano oil in an extra virgin olive oil base.

A highly aromatic Mediterranean oregano oil (blue and yellow label) is the ideal rub for activating thymic function. This works greatly for sick children or pets. In extreme cases where there is sluggish immunity this spice oil should be rubbed routinely at night over the thymus reflexes, which are along the sternum (breast bone) at its intersection with the clavicles. This will greatly strengthen immunity and aid in the fight against chronic conditions, particularly chronic infections. Also, in an extra virgin olive oil base wild oregano oil can be taken internally, two to three drops twice daily. In addition, in the event of radiation exposure the aromatic juice of wild oregano (steam-distilled extract), should be consumed, a half ounce daily. This would help activate and cleanse the immune system.

This oil and juice are true wild spice extracts. Thus, they are safe for all ages. The intake of such extracts is surely necessary, since the immune systems of modern people are heavily burdened with toxic chemicals, poisonous food additives, fungi, and heavy metals. Also, vaccinations devastate immune function, creating a vast burden upon the thymus and, in fact, all the organ systems. Here, natural-source vitamin C made from wild camu camu plus acerola and rose hips is also highly protective.

Chapter Three

How Hormones Work

The endocrine glands are highly specialized. Their key function is to maintain the state of balance within the body. Thus, they are in constant operation in a kind of cooperative symphony with daily life. There is significant strain upon them. Thus, they are always in need of support. As a unit these glands are known as the endocrine system. They are called a system, because they work together as a unit. The function of one gland significantly affects the others. Like a sports team the actions of one directly impact the entire unit. Thus, if one is out of balance, the entire system is disrupted.

This connection must be emphasized. The endocrine glands are links in the same chain. No single part can be affected without all being influenced. The total action of these glands is to keep the body in a fine balance. This is for a wide range of functions, including circulation, resistance to stress, blood sugar control, proper digestion, muscular strength, metabolism, normal mood, balanced immunity, and normal reproduction. It is in order to cause all such functions to operate optimally. This is known as "normal physiology." It is rare.

It might surprise many people how the hormone system works. The various hormone glands are highly delicate and are readily influenced by the slightest degree of stress or toxicity. A single hormone never operates independently. The hormone system operates in an unfathomable balance. There is a natural control, which the various hormones exert. According to *Dorland's Medical Dictionary* a hormone is a "chemical substance, produced in the body...which has a specific regulatory effect..." If the body produces sufficient amounts of such hormones, certainly, regulation will be normal. The symphony within the cells and organs will operate, without missing a note. Thus, the system would be totally intact. This is truly rare. Nearly always there is at least one and usually several endocrine glands which are out of balance.

The whole purpose of the hormones is to influence the function of human cells. They aim to influence the entire body, not merely one isolated portion. There are many other organs or glands in the body which have far less systemic influence than do these hormone-producing organs. The endocrine glands are unique. They operate directly through the blood. This is through their specific secretions, which they dump directly into the bloodstream. This is how they influence the entire body. Once there, the blood carries these secretions to all cells.

Yet, ultimately, relatively little is known about hormone chemistry. This is why this book describes natural ways to balance the endocrine system, rather, to cause it to find its own balance. Tuttle notes in *Textbook of Physiology* that on the cellular level little if anything is known about how these substances work. This is an incredible statement, that after years of research humans are ignorant about how hormones truly work.

So, how can potent hormonal drugs be given? Obviously, these will greatly disrupt this delicate system. Synthetically produced drugs cause corruptions. Such drugs always create imbalances, since, again, no one knows for sure how the endocrine system operates. Only naturally occurring hormones or hormone-boosting agents—the agents made by the almighty creator in perfect chemistry—can be relied upon for major regenerative action. In fact, such agents gently induce a balance in the endocrine system. Then, knowing which natural substances to take, as well as which nutrients are needed to feed the glands, is based upon scientifically discovering the endocrine type. This method is superior to drugs and surgery. In other words, the goal is to balance and nourish the glands, which is achieved through this plan.

There is no need to use drugs for the cure. Food and whole food supplements are sufficiently powerful to normalize the glands. Hormones are found throughout nature. They are found in every plant and animal. Even flowers contain them, and these hormones are relatively potent. Bees collect such hormones by eating the nectar and collecting pollen. These hormones are concentrated in bee products such as pollen, honey, and royal jelly.

According to Fritz Kahn, M.D., throughout nature hormones can be found. For instance, certain flower blossoms contain a hormone very similar to ovarian hormones. Some forms of kelp, namely bull kelp, are particularly high in hormones. Incredibly, such seaweed is rich in a hormone similar to thyroid hormone. He further notes that, like vitamins, hormones are active in unimaginably tiny quantities. This is the power of the biologically synthesized hormones, the ones made in nature by almighty God. These hormones are both safe and effective for endocrine system balancing. So, in fact, such whole foods are effective hormone supplements. Plus, in contrast to drugs they are completely safe for all ages. They are even safe in pregnancy.

The most potent chemicals known

The endocrine balance in the body is subtle. For instance, through their hormones the adrenal glands exert a potent influence on every cell in the body. Yet, incredibly, a year's production is hardly a thirtieth of an ounce. This is a mere gram. This is an incredible fact proving, again, the danger of potent synthetic hormones, which clearly upset the balance in this delicate system. Plus, it proves the importance of balancing the endocrine glands with natural substances, including natural-source hormones, pre-hormones, essential fatty acids, vitamins, and minerals.

Again, consider the delicate yet intensive nature of these glands. Kahn notes that in an entire lifetime the adrenal glands produce only a few tablespoonfuls of hormones. Thus, since their reserve is miniscule only a minimal amount of stress or toxicity is needed to corrupt their function. The fact is despite the powerful influence these glands exert upon the body they are among the most delicate and refined of all organs. The point is their function can be readily disrupted. Then, too, this function can also readily be put into balance. This is through the intake of natural substances which support the hormone system. These substances include royal jelly, bee pollen, kelp, seaweed, crude pumpkinseed oil, crude sesame oil, purple maca, rosemary, sage, wild chaga mushroom, fatty fish oils, particularly wild sockeye salmon oil, wild-like plant fatty acids, such as the critical sacha inchi oil, flower essences, and raw honey. Other herbs/substances which boost hormonal health include lavender, fennel, anise, neroli orange, black (nigella) seed, and fenugreek.

The actions of various hormones differ extensively. So do their biological structures. There is no way to treat such a complex mechanism with synthetic substances. This includes synthetic hormones.

The hormones are found everywhere in the body. Of course, they are highly concentrated in the glands but are also found in the blood, lymph, digestive tract, as well as within the cells. Hormones control the various vital functions, including growth, nutrition, sexual activities, digestion, and nutrition. They also influence brain activity, exerting a direct influence upon mental stamina. They deal with stress, and, of course, stress depletes them. Even personality may be determined by hormonal status. To reiterate, in all the tissues no single hormone acts independently. Rather, the hormones work together to help the body maintain a balance.

Larson in his book *Why We Are What We Are* says that it is virtually impossible to have perfect hormone balance. In other words, regardless of the disease or condition—regardless of how healthy a person truly believes he is—there are always imbalances. If excellent endocrine health is common, notes Larson, "there will be a balanced chemistry, resulting in perfect metabolism, normal function.., and perfect health.." Even in the 1930s, he says, such perfect health was "a rare thing." The fact is the endocrine glands are easily disrupted, even by something as common as food additives in the diet or refined sugar, or perhaps, synthetic perfumes, polluted air/water. It takes little to disrupt them, especially in people with weakened constitutions. This is why perfect balance in modern society is so rare. There are simply too many toxins to deal with, and it is the endocrine system which must process such poisons. What's more, even the naturally occurring poisons, the ones made by body metabolism, are toxic to the endocrine glands. In fact, the endocrine glands are precisely the system which must deal with such toxins. Furthermore, methods for detoxification—for clearing—are a major part of the endocrine treatment plan.

Larson lists the main causes of endocrine imbalance, which are overeating, eating the wrong kinds of foods or wrong combinations of foods, natural toxins produced within the body (from overeating), and, particularly, mental imbalances, including worry, physical strain, and overwork. He also lists lack of exercise as having a highly negative effect upon these glands, as well as harmful habits, such as the intake of drugs, particularly recreational drugs and alcohol.

Alcohol is a decided endocrine poison. Even wine is poisonous to these glands, because any source of alcohol is toxic to them. In particular, the adrenal glands are direly poisoned by alcohol, as is, the pituitary.

Alcohol is a by-product of microbial metabolism. Thus, it is a metabolic poison. Why humans consume it is unexplainable. It is used by bacteria, actually, secreted by them to kill any competitors. In particular, it is highly toxic to rapidly reproducing cells, especially the cells of the liver, stomach, testes, and ovaries. No wonder the regular consumption of this substance causes destruction of such organs. Thus, it is no surprise that the consumption of alcoholic beverages is a major cause of infertility and impotence.

The excessive intake of tea and coffee is also mentioned by Larson as a potential source of toxicity. This is due to the stimulants found in these beverages. These stimulants irritate the glands. Whenever a human overloads his/her body with irritants and/or stimulants, it is the endocrine glands which must attempt to restore balance. Thus, obviously, people create all sorts of strains upon this system as a result of dietary or social excesses. In particular, Larson mentions toxins produced after eating as a major factor in endocrine disruption. The toxins which accumulate as a result of the normal digestion and processing of food greatly burden the endocrine glands, since these glands must constantly work to attempt to restore balance.

These toxins must be cleansed from the body. Once they are cleansed, endocrine balance is restored. After cleansing such toxins from the tissue there is usually a dramatic improvement in body function, which is manifested by an increase in energy and vitality as well as weight loss or in the case of an excessively thin person, weight gain. Undoubtedly, extreme exhaustion is a warning sign of toxin-induced imbalances in these glands. All this supports the value of fasting, which will be discussed later in this book.

It is unnecessary to take energy pills. To gain energy the toxins must be purged. This is through the intake of combinations of wild herbs, wild greens, and spice oils in an extra virgin olive oil, remote-source black seed oil, and apple cider vinegar base. Also, wild berry extracts made from raw, unheated, wild and hand-picked berries are invaluable, particularly for purging the blood and intestines. Wild raw triple greens extracts can also be used.

Note: such cleansing systems are actually gentle and can be taken without compromising lifestyle. They work by purging the inside of cells, as well as the ducts and cells of the liver and the kidneys, not through any laxative effect. There is also a formula for purging consisting of wild raw greens, raw black seed oil, raw extra virgin olive oil, and various spice oils (that is the total body purging system). This greatly eases the pressure on the hormone system. Then, the endocrine glands must be supported nutritionally and hormonally in a natural way. This natural way includes cleansing the body of all toxins which harm the endocrine glands.

The function of the endocrine system is broad. It covers such a wide range of functions that it must be deemed the most critical system known for body regulation. The following is a partial list of the many key functions of the various endocrine hormones:

- maintenance of muscle tone and strength
- production of cellular energy
- mineral (especially calcium) deposition into bones and teeth
- combating allergic reactions
- fighting infection
- combating toxic exposure
- maintenance of normal skin tone and beauty
- maintenance of ideal body shape
- blood sugar regulation
- regulation of blood flow
- maintenance of proper heart function
- digestion and processing of food
- combating inflammation

The metabolic actions of thyroid hormones

Thyroid hormones control much of the body's organ systems. These hormones have a direct effect on virtually all cells and organs of the body. The creation of energy within the body is mainly under thyroid control. The body metabolizes food into energy. In fact, it burns it, much like a car engine burns gasoline. The car engine relies upon the gasoline, made from carbon atoms, to generate energy to 'drive' the car. The human body through its billions of cells relies upon food carbon, that is the carbon molecules of sugar and/or fat atoms, to generate its energy. Thus, all foods that are consumed are processed as a result of the actions of these hormones. This means that hormones control the final processing—the ultimate burning—of food.

The thyroid hormone known as thyroxine, controls the rate of reactions within cells. These are the reactions of combustion. It is responsible for how thoroughly the body uses oxygen. It is also responsible for the creation of heat, for instance, the heat given off during cold weather. In fact, in general exposure to cold activates this gland, while exposure to heat diminishes it.

Cell growth, such as the key growth spurts of infants and children, is thyroid hormone-dependent. Yet, all cells require it as a growth factor, even into old age. For nerves to fire their components must be activated by thyroid hormone. For the heart to pump in ideal rhythm and power this hormone must be present. It is also required for the pumping force, known as the ejection fraction, of this muscle. Thus, in the deficiency a wide range of 'metabolic defects' of the heart and circulation may occur. The ultimate processing of food, its conversion to energy, is dependent upon this hormone. Thus, in the deficiency the metabolism of all categories of foodstuffs, proteins, carbohydrates/sugars, lipids (cholesterol), and fatty acids, is compromised. Here, its influence is vast, since it controls nerve firing, blood circulation, heart rhythm and pumping, cholesterol metabolism, fat burning, sugar/starch burning, vitamin chemistry, and protein synthesis. No wonder the thyroid gland is known as the "Master of Metabolism."

Thyroid hormone is an enzyme activator. The enzymes are proteins, which are, essentially, living entities. Their purpose is to accelerate cellular reactions. When thyroid hormone is lacking, enzyme activity is low. This leads to a reduction in the synthesis of important molecules such as neurotransmitters, hormones, and cell proteins. All cell synthesis, as well as cell repair, is enzyme-dependent. Therefore, all the critical activities within the cell are thyroid hormone-dependent. Enzymes control the speed of how the cells of the body work. Plus, the enzymes are controlled by thyroid hormone.

The enzymes are needed for producing the various proteins needed by the body. There is always a natural wear and tear occurring in all organs. It is the enzymes which stimulate tissue repair. This entire process is under the control of thyroid hormone. No wonder virtually all functions, including digestion, wound healing, circulation, regeneration, and elimination, are impaired when this hormone is lacking.

Thyroid hormone: metabolic giant

When the thyroid hormones are lacking or if the gland is out of balance, it is difficult to metabolize carbohydrates. When foods, such as grains, potatoes, pasta, sugary snacks, bread, rolls, pastries, and even in some instances natural fruit sugars, are consumed rather than being burned, as would be the normal physiology, they are transformed into fat. This fat accumulates first in the liver. Once the liver is overloaded with fat globules the fat/adipose cells are filled. Then, ultimately, the fat may be stored under the skin, often as cellulite. In this imbalance it is simply impossible to burn the carbohydrates fast enough to prevent them from being deposited as fat. Weight gain will continue, as long as the carbohydrates are eaten. In order to halt the weight gain a strict diet must be followed, largely eliminating starchy and sugary foods.

Fruit might be allowed, since it is metabolized rather quickly. However, for people with weak thyroid glands it cannot be eaten in vast quantities. Usually, the hypothyroid individual must be restricted to rather low-sugar fruit such as melon, limes, lemons, grapefruit, kiwi fruit, strawberries, blueberries, and papayas. Fruit high in sugar, particularly apples, pears, oranges, peaches, cherries, and grapes, should be avoided. Dried fruit and fruit juices should be avoided or at least restricted. Fruit juices made from low-sugar fruit, such as tomato, pomegranate, blueberry, cranberry, papaya, and grapefruit juice, can be consumed. Occasionally, freshly squeezed orange juice, cut 50/50 with grapefruit juice, is tolerated. Thus, since such individuals are unable to metabolize carbohydrates, restricting such calories is a simple cure.

In hypothyroidism the synthesis, as well as digestion, of protein is also impaired. Recall that when thyroid hormone is lacking the enzyme systems fail. This includes the all-important digestive enzymes such as those secreted by the stomach and pancreas. Such enzymes are required for splitting apart the proteins from food, converting them into amino acids.

Without good enzyme activity the absorption of protein is severely compromised. Always, in hypothyroidism the enzyme activity is reduced. Thus, the amount of protein available in the blood is diminished. This is particularly dangerous relative to the heart, lungs, and circulation. This is because in order to maintain blood and fluid volume protein is necessary. A lack of protein may lead to a wide range of disorders, including congestive heart failure, swelling in the extremities, thick swellings under the skin (myxedema), kidney disorders, joint damage, immune deficiency, and liver disease.

The liver is also highly dependent upon protein. Without it, liver cells readily degenerate. Researchers have found that in hypothyroidism the liver cells make protein grudgingly. In extreme protein deficiency the liver becomes permanently damaged, a condition known as cirrhosis. Here is the dilemma: a person with sluggish thyroid function may eat enough protein for their body's needs, however, he or she is unable to metabolize it. In extreme cases of hypothyroidism liver function fails, that is cirrhosis. If the condition is resolved, thyroid function is restored. This is only if the liver regenerates. Otherwise, there will be a degree of hypothyroidism, because of the fact that it is the liver which activates this hormone.

Thyroid hormone not only burns fat, but it also helps regulate the metabolism as well as synthesis of critical fats. The entire metabolism of cholesterol is dependent upon it. In fact, a high cholesterol level is a key marker for thyroid hormone deficiency. It tells of sluggish metabolism. It means that fats or, more correctly, lipids are building up in the blood. This is because when the thyroid is defective, glucose can't be burned. So, the body converts this sugar into fats and/or cholesterol. Sometimes, this is represented by fatty cholesterol deposits in the face as well as the arteries. A person with yellowish waxy deposits under and around the eyes likely suffers from hypothyroidism, in fact, this is virtually assured. These deposits are known as xanthomas.

In women with mildly to moderately elevated cholesterol plus slight or significant weight problems rather than cardiac pathology the first consideration is a metabolic disorder, that is the problem of sluggish thyroid function. Incredibly, hundreds of thousands of women, as well as men, are rushed into hospitals or doctors' offices for invasive cardiovascular testing—and even surgery—when the problem is exclusively metabolic. Had a careful history been taken, along with the appropriate blood tests, the true diagnosis could be found, and expensive and even dangerous procedures could be avoided.

While it is little recognized most of the cholesterol made in the body is used as part of the digestive process. It is consumed in the formation of bile, the latter being required for fat digestion. This is another connection of thyroid hormone to digestion. This hormone is needed to convert cholesterol to bile acids. Thus, when the hormone is lacking, fat digestion stalls. This is a vicious cycle; the cholesterol fails to be metabolized, which impairs fat digestion. As a result, it accumulates in the blood, causing blockages. If the thyroid function is boosted, the cholesterol deposits are mobilized, in fact, cleansed.

Thyroid hormone also directly acts upon fat cells. Actually, it helps activate a fat-burning mechanism within them. This is far from claiming that thyroid hormone will induce weight loss. However, it is certain that a lack of thyroid hormone interferes with fat burning. Thus, to stimulate weight loss the key is to normalize thyroid function, so that fat can be burned efficiently. It works best if combined with adrenal therapy and, in women, natural therapy for the ovaries. B vitamins also increase the efficiency of thyroid hormones and are, certainly, required for their activation. Here, niacin and thiamine are particularly essential. Even a mild lack of either of these vitamins results in thyroid gland dysfunction.

Even vitamin chemistry is under the control of this hormone. Thyroid hormone converts, for instance, the B vitamins from food or inert forms into biologically active ones. Thus, hypothyroid individuals may suffer from severe vitamin deficiencies, even if they receive sufficient amounts in their diets. They simply are unable to convert the vitamins into the usable forms. So, even though they consume sufficient amounts, they develop vitamin deficiency symptoms, often to the extreme. This is because rather than simply a deficiency, it is a metabolic defect with which they are afflicted. They may even take potent vitamin supplements and still be deficient. Vitamins which are dependent upon thyroid hormone for proper activation include thiamine, niacin, riboflavin, vitamin B_6, vitamin C, coenzyme Q-10, and vitamin A. The key to correcting these deficiencies is to achieve balanced thyroid function. However, it may be necessary to supplement the diet with these nutrients.

Riboflavin is found naturally in rich amounts in a wild triple greens flush. Here, a mere ounce of this wild raw greens extract contains a milligram. This is an exceedingly high amount for this rare natural vitamin. Even small amounts of such wild greens, like 40 drops daily, will help replenish riboflavin stores. Also, this vitamin is found in a wild greens beverage, known as Super-5-Greens (see Americanwildfoods.com). The vitamin is also found in dense amounts in undiluted royal jelly, either as a paste or lyophilized capsules, as well as torula yeast. It is unnecessary to take huge amounts. Microdoses will suffice to keep the balance. This nutrient is also found in rich supplies in organic liver, kidney, and heart.

In the case of niacin the best natural sources are rice bran, rice polish, and undiluted royal jelly. Wild rice is also an excellent source. For vitamin A the true natural vitamin A from fatty fish liver is ideal. The two best sources of vitamin A are cod liver oil and unprocessed sockeye salmon oil. Both these oils are from wild fish. Beta carotene supplements should be avoided, since hypothyroid individuals are usually unable to convert this vegetable form of vitamin A into its animal or active form.

Ultimately, natural-source vitamins are superior to the synthetic types. For supplements with natural-source vitamins see the makers of rice bran/polish-based powders, tropical fruit-source vitamin C, 3x royal jelly, remote-source purple corn, crude cold-pressed pumpkinseed oil, crude cold-pressed sesame seed oil, crude red sour grape (as a source of chromium), crude wild oregano (as a source of calcium, magnesium, and phosphorus), crude wild greens in a raw state (as a source of riboflavin), and similar supplements.

There is also a natural-source vitamin C in the form of wild camu camu plus rose hips and acerola. A truly natural crude vitamin E derived from sunflower seed oil, with crude red palm oil and pumpkinseed oil is also available.

It is best to always opt for natural vitamins and minerals versus the synthetic, since the natural types are the only ones proven safe and truly effective.

Metabolism for life: the role of the adrenal glands

The adrenal glands are the body's coping system. They are also the key system for producing antiinflammatory compounds. The adrenal glands deal with all sorts of stress, psychological as well as physical. They also produce hormones for metabolizing carbohydrates.

There is a direct connection between the brain and the adrenal glands. This is through the spinal cord and also through the pituitary. Thus, mental pressure has a direct impact on the adrenals, disrupting the flow of adrenal hormones. The adrenal glands also make adrenalin (as the name indicates), which is an anti-stress hormone. This is the inner part of these organs, known as the medulla. Here, the focus will be on the hormones made by the outer part, or cortex.

Unlike other parts of these glands, notes Best and Taylor in *Physiological Basis of Medical Practice*, the cortex is "essential to life." Even removal of only about two-thirds of the organs can result in sudden death. Yet, only ten percent of the liver is needed or half or less of a kidney for survival. This means that other than the heart and brain the adrenals are the most critical organs for survival.

These glands make an enormous variety of hormones, more than all the rest of the endocrine glands combined. Some 60 different hormones are produced by the adrenal glands, including cortisone, progesterone, aldosterone,

DHEA, estrogen, and testosterone. Thus, it is no surprise that the adrenal glands support the function of the reproductive glands.

Deficiency of adrenal hormones has been well researched. In the extreme there is tiredness and muscle weakness. Digestion is disturbed. Here, there is often a vague kind of indigestion that defies diagnosis. There may be diarrhea and/or constipation, or this may alternate. There can be spastic colitis. Body temperature is usually low, and the skin is clammy; there is sensitivity to extremes in temperature. Neck pain and stiffness is common, as is pain and/or aching in the mid-to-upper back. A persistent ache in the mid-to-lower back may even indicate infection of the adrenal glands, notably by tubercular germs. However, in extreme cases exhaustion is the most notable symptom, along with the inability to concentrate. The exhaustion itself may be a sign of TB. Regardless, such extreme cases are also represented by a bronzing of the skin or pigment spots about the temples.

The adrenal glands are involved in virtually all body processes. They are crucial for blood sugar regulation. Here, they are involved with causing the liver to produce a storage form of glucose, known as glycogen. Salt and water metabolism is also under adrenal control. This relates to blood volume. In fact, the maintenance of this blood volume is virtually exclusively an adrenal function. This blood volume is essential to the function of the heart. It is a function of salt retention in the bloodstream, which is a function of these glands. This is why heart attacks and congestive heart failure may be primarily adrenal diseases. In the adequate treatment of these diseases it is essential that the adrenal component is considered.

People with weak adrenals likely have a condition known as hypoglycemia. In this condition blood sugar levels are not properly maintained. Much sugar is used by the brain. Thus, many of the symptoms of this condition involve the brain and nerves, including depression, irritability, anxiety, panic attacks, agitation, moodiness, and temper tantrums. The muscular system also needs glucose. Thus, other symptoms of this condition include muscle spasms, leg cramps, stiff neck, stiff upper back, and muscle twitching. Headaches are also a common manifestation of low blood sugar. This may explain why this symptom is common in people with adrenal dysfunction.

The sex glands: human power plants?

The sex organs play a major role in overall health, not merely the sex act. These glands are responsible for creating a lively personality. To a large degree they give men and women their physical power. The charisma of a person can be due to the hormones produced by these glands. Without these hormones, vitality, in fact, strength is lost.

If such glands are damaged or destroyed or if they are removed surgically, the human 'sexual' power-base is lost. To a large degree these organs control fat deposition. This is particularly true in women. Excellently functioning ovaries largely prevent fat accumulation. If the ovaries are weak, this negatively affects the thyroid, reducing the metabolic rate. As a result, fat is readily deposited, since in the event of ovarian insufficiency the body has difficulty converting food into fuel. Rather, the fuel in the form of sugars is converted into fat instead of being burned into energy within the cells. Both thyroid and ovarian hormones are needed to activate such cellular burning. Thus, weak ovaries are a major cause of obesity.

The sex glands become developed mostly before 20 years of age. The master gland in their development is the pineal and to a lesser degree the pituitary. If these glands are weak or diseased, the sex glands will mature poorly. Of note zinc and protein deficiency may greatly impair the functions of these glands. Zinc deficiency is notable by the existence of white spots on the fingernails. Protein deficiency may be noted by puffiness and/or swelling in the body. Curiously, multiple white spots on the nails are commonly seen in thyroid types. This tells of malabsorption of zinc, which of course will impair thyroid function. These spots may also reveal intolerance to wheat, since the gluten in this grain readily destroys the absorptive surface of the intestines, leading to zinc malabsorption.

Most doctors believe that it is the pituitary which controls sex gland development. However, it was Larson who again determined that it is primarily the pineal that is responsible, the pituitary being a distant second. Between the two, the pineal and pituitary, sexual development is determined. Thus, it is organs in the brain which are directly responsible for sexual development. This may explain why people with mental disorders often have underdeveloped sex glands. Too, the urge for sex is largely generated in the brain. People create the sexual urge through their thoughts. Thus, it is not a surprise that people who are mentally retarded are also retarded in their sexual powers.

Sexual power is far from evil, if it is channeled in a positive direction. This is in the form of true and natural love. It only becomes evil if it is mis-channeled.

A weak constitution is never respected. A powerful constitution is admired, in fact, envied. A powerful man is the envy of all. In certain societies powerful women are admired. The key with male or female hormone energy is to channel it in the right direction. It is the wrong direction to use it as a "conquering force" to abuse others. It is the right direction to channel it into physical and mental power. This is through using it to create presence. That is how to take the greatest advantage of this energy.

It is possible to be sexually powerful, without violating the rules of common decency. Thus, it is important for the human race to build the strength of the sex glands through proper nourishment and natural hormonal support. This is far from the purpose of merely being strong or virile during the sex act. Rather, it is for the health of the overall chemistry, physique, and beauty. It is for the vitality that healthy glandular function provides. It is never for the purpose of proving sexual vigor to the detriment of others.

Persons with a weakened pineal-sex gland connection are often physically weak. Such individuals tire easily. This is even after minimal exertion. They have minimal or no sex drive. Often, they are frumpy in appearance, with poor muscle tone. For women sagging features are common. Often, there is little or no libido, and it takes enormous stimulation to create desire. This is their tendency. It is not due to mental or psychological problems. They are weak hormonally, which makes them weak sexually. Perhaps this is a natural medicine, as people with feeble pituitary/pineal function are often too weak to properly raise children. This is typical of the pituitary type, as described later in the book. It is also typical of people with genetic defects.

Chapter Four

The Symphony in Action

For ideal health the discovery of the hormonal weakness is crucial. This is the answer to the majority of health problems. Metabolism can vary greatly in different individuals. This is under hormonal control. This is why each person must know his/her type. People could even be from the same family, and their metabolism could differ drastically. Everyone is different. That's how God made it.

The hormone type is the key to health improvement. This is perhaps the most useful tool for quickly boosting overall health. This is because proper treatment is dependent on the nature of the metabolism. So is the diet.

A person could collapse, develop a disease, virtually die of allergic reactions, or even die prematurely, and it is all unnecessary. Broda Barnes, M.D., proved long ago that sudden death, especially from heart disease, is largely due to an underlying thyroid disorder. Thus, he proved the true danger of hormonal weakness. This high risk is especially true in women. He demonstrated that these deaths were preventable by curing the thyroid dysfunction. Thus, the knowledge of the hormone type is essential for preventing premature death. This makes the hormonal type perhaps the most important personalized health information anyone can acquire.

Knowing the type can help in the reversal of disease. If that metabolism can be enhanced, then, the overall health will improve, as is demonstrated by the following case history:

> Ms. M. is a vivacious and cheerful 44-year-old. However, her health was a challenge. Despite being a nutritionist she was plagued with chronic shortness of breath for which she in the past took medication. She was also sluggish in the morning but active at night. She complained to a degree of brain fogginess. Also, she had just endured a prolonged case of respiratory distress, which was still unresolved. Analysis revealed she was a thyroid type, with a kind of rectangular face and drooping cheeks. Her index finger was shorter than the ring. However, her frame was medium and she wasn't heavy.
>
> After analyzing her I suggested she begin eating pure seafood, avoid all soy, and take a special supplement made from high-grade remote-source northern Pacific kelp plus wild oregano, rosemary, and tyrosine. She was also given oil of wild oregano to purge fungus. This was all she was given, but it was based upon a careful analysis of her type. After taking the supplements, within 24 hours her breathing massively improved. She felt a wellness she had not experienced in 20 years.

So, the key is to start with discovering the individual metabolism. Then, correct treatment must be taken. This may also prevent the greatest of all crises, which is premature death. It can also prevent medical disasters, that is the disaster of receiving the wrong medical treatment or dangerous medical procedures, all because no attempt was made to discover the cause, which is faulty metabolism. Innumerable surgeries and drug prescriptions are administered for no good reason and without cure, in fact, to the patient's detriment. It is simply because the metabolic/hormonal status was never evaluated.

The power of metabolism

There are no exceptions to this rule, that is this existence of unique metabolic status. This unique metabolic status is the key to discovering the correct therapy.

The priority is to determine a person's endocrine or metabolic status. This is because adjustments in such a pattern could prove highly valuable. Such adjustments could mean the difference between the onset of disease and its prevention. It is also the means to reverse existing disease. What's more, in those who are unable to cope or who are tired or weak proper endocrine balancing will rapidly reverse symptoms. People pursue a wide range of means to improve health, including diet, exercise, attitude improvement, and spiritual advancement. Yet, the key way to achieve optimal health is to take into account the rate of individualized metabolism. Then, this metabolism must be normalized through natural therapies. It is this factor alone which is responsible for the rapid return of health as well as its precipitous decline.

Think about it. What are the consequences of stress, which are exclusively mediated through this system? The brain and nerves are merely end organs. They are somewhat mechanical, rather, electrical. It is the thoughts which influence the brain. Then, it is the endocrine glands which control the way the brain and nerves respond. For instance, what happens during a fear reaction? The entire body descends into disarray. This results in the outpouring of endocrine secretions, which create the "fight or flight" response. What about being confronted by a hostile worker or even a thief, mugger, or rapist? Then, what of the person in the midst of war, shell-shocked and traumatized? Again, these glands bear the consequences. This explains why people who are mugged or raped seemingly never completely recover from the trauma. They develop a kind of fright syndrome. The toxic memory is retained and continues to cause distress at the slightest fear. This is an endocrine response, the memory for which is stored in the nervous system.

In today's fast-paced world all people suffer a certain degree of distress. People who manage this are in the most optimal health. Yet, the existence of a perfect endocrine/metabolic status is unknown. This is especially true in today's age. There are several major factors accounting for this lack of perfection. These factors include poor diet, the ubiquitous nature of synthetic toxins, which deplete endocrine function, nutritional deficiency, a high complex of refined carbohydrates, and mental duress. So, in modern life no one has perfect endocrine function. At a minimum there are too many social stresses, plus the quality of food is in decline. A perfect lifestyle with plenty of relaxation, ease, comfort, sunshine, fresh air, and pure food is required to have perfect glandular function. Who in this world achieves this?

The metabolic glands are far from isolated structures. These glands are involved directly in all affairs of the body. Centrally located, they guide the most critical functions. They do so through a unified approach. Despite this, doctors treat the endocrine glands independently, that is as an isolated system. Thus, they never consider the role played by their fellows. In medicine this isolation treatment does more harm than good.

In medical textbooks these glands are regarded separately. Little if anything is mentioned about their vast interconnections. Even so, a defect in one, incredibly, impacts the entire system. Yet, to isolate the glands—to treat them as separate organs—is disastrous. Doctors treat these organs with aggressive drugs, which disrupts the entire system. Again, within the body all glands work as a unit. If one gland is out of tune, it disrupts the entire mechanism. The other glands must compensate. Thus, if any of the components are disturbed, the system is weakened. This is important to understand, because it is the basis of appropriate treatment. This is the intake of the proper diet plus food concentrates versus single or synthetic hormones. It is also the use of herbs and essential oils.

If the stress is continuous and/or if the imbalance fails to be corrected, the entire system becomes dysfunctional. Moreover, since all the endocrine glands are interconnected, treatment should always consider this. Isolated treatment produces minimal or temporary effects. Rather, such treatment disrupts the mechanism, usually causing irreparable damage. Thus, the objective should be to devise a coordinated effort aimed at balancing the entire system. This will produce the greatest results.

It was again Larson who claimed that while a state of perfection in the anatomy and size of the endocrine glands is rare, even if these glands were perfect there are always stresses, which create upsets. This is how life works regarding people who are exposed to events, stresses, and toxicities, which distress the organism. The degree of distress depends largely upon how a person handles any challenges. Those who mentally become distressed or worry greatly suffer from depleted endocrine reserve. In contrast, those who take a more upbeat approach, knowing that they can control or minimize their reactions, that is through the proper attitude, fair better. They tend to retain much of their reserve. Even so, most people living in the Western world, especially Americans, suffer from depleted endocrine reserve. What's more, the more they worry the more greatly depleted it becomes. Yet, they can use a positive approach to, in fact, build it up. Happiness builds endocrine strength. Worry and frustration, as well as sadness, exhaust it. So, strong people—that is people who always remain positive and refuse to worry—have a powerful endocrine reserve.

With endocrine health attitude is the key. People can control their metabolism through their attitudes. All people experience challenges. It is how the individual handles the challenges which determines the metabolic consequences. Grief, depression, and agitation greatly damage the glands. Yet, with a mere change in attitude this can be quickly reversed. To reverse this it is only necessary to change the thought pattern. Here, in particular the adrenals are highly responsive. Positive emotions produce steroids, which are mood enhancing. Peace and serenity heal these glands.

The endocrine system is easily disrupted. Any serious accident or disease greatly destabilizes glandular function.

Poor diet and the intake of stimulants also disturbs function. Thus, a person with strong, healthy endocrine glands can develop dysfunctional glands due to trauma, sickness, or abusive habits. Drugs also disrupt the glands and can rapidly destabilize them. However, if the drugs are eliminated and/or illnesses purged, the glands may rapidly heal. Even so, prolonged or repeated use of cortisone and/or prednisone creates vast damage, especially to the adrenal glands. However, as long as the damage or toxicity remains the endocrine glands will remain disturbed.

Prolonged illness may result in permanent damage. True, the endocrine glands can regenerate. Even so, this can only occur to a degree. There will always be some wear and tear. Without constantly attempting to build the health of these glands there will be a degree of damage, a sort of 'toxic' aging. This is because the endocrine glands are the human's coping mechanism. If the body is freed of illness, this releases the endocrine glands of their strenuous duties. As a result, these glands may readily recover. Yet, to achieve this recovery, often, much support is needed. This can be accomplished through radical changes in the diet and the elimination of stimulants and poisons plus the intake of nutritional supplements.

Certain vitamin-mineral supplements may also be needed. In fact, unless the imbalances in the endocrine system are corrected the achievement of excellent health remains illusive. There may well be other issues to resolve such as chronic infections, solvent intoxication, and heavy metal toxicity. Yet, these, too, are related to the endocrine damage. Infections, along with heavy metal toxicity, destabilize endocrine function. These toxicities must be resolved for the endocrine system to be freed from its depression. This emphasizes the need for natural substances which help purge the body of toxins as well as infections. Such substances include oil of wild oregano (hand-picked, Mediterranean), wild raw greens complex, a purging system based upon extra virgin olive oil, black seed oil, wild spice oils, and wild berry as well as greens extracts. This is a total system purge. For this to be effective it must be in a raw state. This combination is a powerful purge for reducing the stress upon the hormone glands. Such cleansing is critical for regenerating endocrine function.

The mind, infection, and more

The mental state is a reflection of endocrine health. Again, the brain is largely controlled by the endocrine glands. In fact, if the hypothalamus is included, the status of the endocrine glands is virtually fully responsible for mood. All endocrine activity begins in the brain, but it is not just for the rest of the body. These brain-based glands also make hormones, which influence the brain itself. Plus, these hormones direct the function of the lower glands: the adrenals, thyroid, liver, pancreas, thymus, parathyroid, testes, and ovaries. Without the cerebral connection there is no activity in the glands. Yet, as mentioned previously the glands within the brain, the pituitary and pineal, also control its metabolism. Thus, in any illness of the brain the influence of the endocrine glands must be considered. Also, the lower glands exert influence over this region through various feed-back mechanisms.

In particular, the adrenal glands and thyroid have a direct effect upon the mental state. Yet, so do the ovaries and testes.

Incredibly, as described by Larson as early as the 1920s, pessimism was regarded as being directly related to the function of the endocrine glands. In men it was found that a reduced output of testicular hormones somehow directly impacts the brain, leading to a negative, pessimistic attitude. This involves the interactions between the testes and the pituitary. Larson describes a connection between the weakened testicular function and the pituitary as well as adrenals. If the function of any of these glands is strengthened, the negativity and pessimism disappear. The pessimism/negativity, he says, can be altered in two ways. This is through proper strengthening of the involved endocrine glands and mental training.

It is possible to train the brain to react positively instead of negatively. Plus, if a person realizes he has the negative tendency, the destructive thoughts can be more readily warded off. Larson claims that, in fact, the pituitary can be strengthened through "constructive and logical thinking and reasoning. This exercise...will develop a powerful pituitary and convert the individual from a pessimist to an ultra-optimist, from a coward to a courageous individual."

It is hormone power which gives strength to the character. True, what a person thinks, rather, what he or she believes, plays a crucial role. Yet, the combination of healthy thinking plus correct nutrition can make the difference between a mentally stable and productive person and human disaster. The role of the mind in glandular health is immense. It is critical to understand this, since pessimism truly is a cause of untold human misery. Good things happen, but only through a positive outlook.

A negative attitude only produces greater negativity. This negativity destructively affects all aspects of a person's life.

Could an athlete win a contest with a negative attitude? This is impossible. Surely, his opponent, who sports a positive attitude, would defeat him. The mind cannot be taught, that is trained, for defeat and yet win. Then, how could anyone win at life, whether in relationships, business, or pleasure—especially while thinking negatively? A negative attitude only leads to despair. Thus, there is only one avenue for superior health. It is to halt all negative thinking before this destructive influence leads to a decline in overall health. People destroy themselves with their thoughts. About this there can be no doubt.

If the nature of a loved one is more well understood, it is possible to be more compassionate about specific differences. If a dear one is different in behavior, emotions, and physiology, that is vitality, be careful of being critical. It isn't the individual's fault. These differences are inherent: they are within his/her natural metabolism.

Chapter Five

The Endocrine Types

The endocrine glands have a vast influence on the body. This is even true of the boney skeleton. It is true of weight patterns, bone density, finger length, and other physical features. There are four major endocrine types. These are the thyroid, adrenal, pituitary, and thyroid-adrenal types. Less common types include the adrenal-thyroid and pituitary-thyroid-adrenal, as well as the thyroid-muscular, the latter also being known as the muscular-pancreatic type.

Endocrine disorders occur most commonly in females. This is because females have the greatest number of endocrine glands. It is also due to the strain upon the glands from pregnancy, childbirth, and nursing. According to W. Engelbach, M.D., in his book *Endocrine Medicine,* in the 1930s the ratio of female to male endocrine disorders was 3:1. However, males are gaining ground. This may largely be the result of pollution with estrogen-like molecules.

A variety of pesticides have estrogenic actions, as do plastics residues. Soy is also estrogenic. Thus, for any woman who suffers from estrogen-dominant diseases, including breast and uterine cancer, the intake of soy must be banned. This is particularly true of genetically engineered soy and its derivatives. These derivatives include GM soy oil, vitamin E, and lecithin.

Birth control pills and estrogen drugs, which are feminizing, have contaminated the waterways. So, when boys or men drink estrogen-contaminated tap water, over time, they can develop feminine characteristics. These estrogenic substances are also absorbed from the soil into the food. Thus, in the United States there is an epidemic of a kind of de-masculization syndrome, where males fail to develop properly. This is surely diet- and pollution-induced.

The endocrine status largely determines a person's power as well as vulnerability. Yet, when a person *controls* the vulnerability, this is how power is gained. Thus, through such a system the individual can find his or her weaknesses and, therefore, determine how to protect the self. For instance, with thyroid types there is a high vulnerability to heart attacks, much higher than the norm. Why suffer such an event, when it is avoidable? If no action is taken, for a thyroid type, especially males, a cardiac event could occur at any time. By taking certain preventive measures the heart attack risk is essentially eliminated. This is by boosting thyroid function with a complex of wild herbs, spices, and northern Pacific kelp. Also, a multiple spice complex, containing extracts of fenugreek, myrtle, cinnamon oleoresin, and cumin, can be taken to eliminate insulin resistance. As well, thyroid types are often infected by fungi, and this infestation must be purged.

With the adrenal type there is also a tendency to develop chronic infections. In particular, there is an unusual propensity for viral lung infections. There is also a high tendency for bacterial lung infections as well as fungal infections of the lungs and bronchial tubes. These are the individuals who readily develop chronic bronchitis and asthma. Incredibly, the adrenal types are also at a high risk for the development of tuberculosis. Here, with weak adrenals the resistance against such subtle, pervasive invaders is virtually nil. This accounts for the finding on autopsy in people who die of adrenal failure of TB infection actually in the glands. The question is does the TB cause the adrenal collapse, or is it an opportunist?

Thus, it becomes apparent that, again, knowledge is empowering. By understanding the attributes and vulnerable aspects of their body types, the individual can take the appropriate precautions.

The shape of the body is a key revelation. Here, the shape of the entire body, plus that of the head, is particularly telling. So are the finger lengths. Symptoms also give evidence of the endocrine/metabolic type. All this will be thoroughly evaluated in order to precisely determine each person's type.

The thyroid type (slow metabolizer)

The thyroid gland exerts a potent influence upon body functions. As stated previously it is known as the "master of metabolism," since it exerts the most crucial role in metabolic rate. This gland exerts a direct effect upon immune function as well as circulation. Also, during growth and development it directly acts upon the critical organ systems, such as the bones, joints, and muscles, spurring normal growth.

The thyroid type may be large- or small-framed. Usually, people of this type often have strong or thick bodies. Yet, this is not always the case. They may be frail or thin-boned. With extreme thyroid disorders much weight is gained, some as fat and some as a kind of protein-rich fluid. This may make these individuals appear big-boned, but they may, in fact, be small-boned. Regardless of the type of frame the treatment is largely the same. Even so, the person with the small-boned type usually also suffers from adrenal weakness. In a small-framed person, who carries large amounts of weight, this is

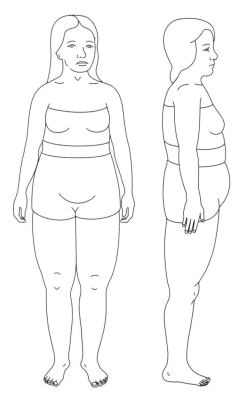

Fig. 1 Female thyroid body type

rarely exclusively a thyroid case. Usually, there is also a pituitary and/or adrenal component, especially if the head is noticeably small for the size of the body. In the true thyroid type the head is normal or large for the size of the body.

Usually, thyroid types are medium-boned. However, the tissues appear unusually thick, even swollen. The contour of the facial bones is often lost. In the extreme the tissues are puffy. The facial tissues often droop or sag. The corners of the eyes droop downward, as do the corners of the mouth. The thick-appearing woman is distinctive. Height is not

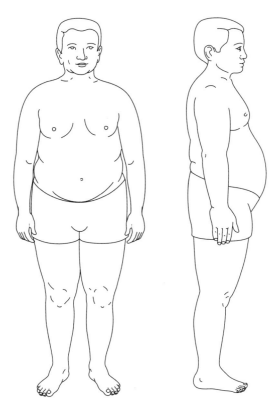

Fig. 2 Male thyroid body type

distinctive. These individuals can be short, although they are usually of medium height.

One prominent feature is the head. In both males and females it is often square. The head may also be rectangular in shape, as is the forehead. In some people with thyroid type it is oval in shape. The body may be square-shaped or rectangular. Although excessive weight is common, a hypothyroid individual may also be of moderate weight. In almost all cases the excess weight is stored in the front of the body, heavily in the front of the abdomen and thighs and less so in the buttocks. In general, in the front they are apple shaped.

Thyroid types are not always grossly fat. The thickness of the tissues, especially the skin, makes them appear obese. Women with pendulous abdomens, swelling in the legs or ankles, and/or elephant-like legs are usually severely hypothyroid.

For some individuals virtually all their dysfunction arises from this gland. True, there must always be other endocrine components, particularly imbalances in the adrenals, ovaries, and pituitary. If the thyroid is out of balance, it is expected that these other glands will also be dysfunctional. In particular, in women a thyroid disorder is certain evidence of ovarian dysfunction.

The key with the thyroid type is balance. Doctors have traditionally treated this gland as an isolated organ, giving potent drugs. True, some of these drugs are naturally derived from beef or pork pancreas. However, the thyroid gland is part of a symphony of endocrine organs. Truly, it operates in unison with all others. Thus, treating a 'thyroid condition' with only the isolated hormone may be counterproductive. It may temporarily resolve many of the symptoms, but the dilemma is if such potent hormones are taken long-term, imbalances may well occur in various other organ systems. Even the thyroid gland may suffer from an imbalance, hopelessly repressed due to the overpowering effects of replacement hormone.

Balance is achieved by feeding it nutritionally. It is also achieved by the intake of natural-source hormones, as well as certain herbs and plant extracts, which boost endocrine function. True, some individuals have no option but to regularly take thyroid drugs due to surgical removal of this

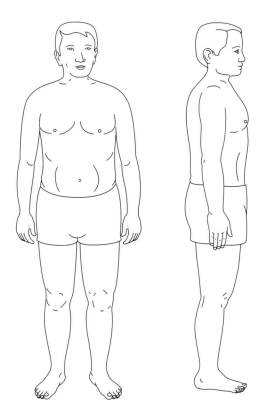

Fig. 3 Male thyroid body type (non-obese version)

gland or its destruction by radioactive iodine. In such cases individuals are essentially thyroid cripples. They must take the hormone or risk serious consequences. However, for all others the ideal treatment is to create a balanced function, where the thyroid produces its own hormones and where it, therefore, is able to function adequately, without medication. Yet, even in extreme cases the proper nutritional and herbal supplement regimen may help normalize the thyroid glands, even, perhaps, without the need for medication.

The delicate balance of this gland and its secretions is demonstrated by the well-known results of taking thyroid drugs. The person may experience nervousness, agitation, sweating, rapid heart beat, heart rhythm disturbances, chest pain and possible digestive disorders. The synthetic version, Synthroid, is associated with osteoporosis, that is bone loss. In particular, with toxic reactions to Synthroid cardiac symptoms may predominate: there may be excessive nervousness as well as skipped beats and palpitations. It is merely that the intake is greater than the usage. Therefore, the hormone accumulates. This agitates the cells. Also, this is only a single hormone, while natural-source thyroid consists of multiple hormones. It is only one molecule in a litany of compounds. Thus, the organ system is thrown out of balance through the regular intake of synthetic thyroid hormone.

Usually, with the synthetic there is no danger, even though rather frightening cardiovascular symptoms may develop. This is because in the vast majority of the cases the patient realizes he or she is taking an excess and, thus, reduces the dose. Only rarely do serious or life-threatening reactions result. Thus, thyroid hormones are among the safest drugs known. Even so, if the thyroid can be balanced naturally without drugs, this is preferable.

It has been presumed that deranged thyroid function is due primarily to iodine deficiency. It has also been established that goiter is directly caused by such a deficiency. It was again Larson in his book *Why We Are What We Are* who takes issue with this. He claims that the blaming of all goiter and/or thyroid conditions on a lack of this substance is fraudulent. He established that weak secretions of the entire endocrine glands, not merely the thyroid, is the cause of goiter. He defines this further by claiming that it is weakness of the secretions during puberty which is the cause. Thus, he proposes, if the endocrine glands could be naturally strengthened during this time, the entire problem of sluggish thyroid and/or goiter would be eliminated.

There is a degree of modern proof for his finding. It is now known that many cases of sluggish thyroid syndrome, as well as goiter, develop in teenagers. It is incredibly common in the United States, that is this occurrence of thyroid problems during the teenager years, even in childhood. Often, a normal or even relatively thin individual suddenly begins to gain weight. Soon, there develops a full-blown thyroid imbalance.

Yet, today, the body simply cannot cope hormonally with the stress of growth. Nutritional deficiency increases the risk. The intake of highly processed foods precipitates it. Larson notes that in such teenagers simply nourishing the glands and providing hormonal supplements normalized the function, usually within the year. He gave no iodine. However, his experience has been recently upgraded, that is through a combined approach. This is because there is often even a greater degree of improvement if good nourishment, hormonal support, and natural iodine sources are combined. With such an approach virtually any childhood or teenage thyroid condition can be cured, without medication.

This entire concept that the endocrine glands are over-taxed and out of balance rather than mere iodine deficiency was based upon early observations. Larson, a surgeon, had many opportunities to observe the causes first-hand. He noticed that while young girls and teenagers had swollen or distressed thyroid glands, this rarely happened in young teenage boys. In examining children he found that it was the females who developed swollen or enlarged thyroids, while with the males the glands remained 'normal.' He describes a family of, for instance, ten children, five females and five males. The females all developed swollen thyroids, while no such deformity occurred in the males. This he attributed to the fact that the females had to contend with the menstrual cycle, which places great stress not only on the thyroid but also upon the ovaries and even the adrenals. Thus, developing girls readily suffer a full-body endocrine deficiency. Combine this stress with the toxicity of a processed food diet and the stage is set for thyroid collapse, since this gland helps control the menstrual process as well as the food metabolism.

By causing these various glands to function in balance Larson cured the thyroid disorders, as well as goiters, even without supplemental iodine. Yet, as will be discussed in Chapter 5, iodine has some value, and it does benefit endocrine function. Thus, the combined approach of iodine-rich foods, healthy diet, and natural iodine supplements plus natural endocrine support for all the glands offers the best and most rapid results. While with Larson's therapy, which primarily involved glandular supplements plus improved diet, the problems were cured over months or years. With the combined approach described in this book, results will be seen within a week or two, and a cure can be expected with a few months or even less.

Even Larson determined that the iodine is critical. It is desperately needed by both the thyroid gland and the ovaries. The ovaries concentrate this mineral, where it stimulates the secretion of female hormones, including estrogen and progesterone. Plus, the ovaries produce their own iodine-based thyroid-like hormone, *diiodotyrosine*. Thus, the thyroid and the ovaries work as a unit, and, therefore, any supportive therapy must take this fact into account. Only by normalizing the function of both glands can sluggish thyroid (that is hypothyroidism), and/or goiter be efficiently cured. What's more, by applying such a treatment the cure will be permanent. In fact, the thyroid-like hormones produced in the ovary have a direct effect upon the thyroid, as well as other female organs, such as the breasts and uterus. This is why in order to correct any supposed thyroid disorder the ovaries must also be treated. Thus, as claimed by Larson "goiter is due to endocrine dysfunction." Rather than a thyroid disorder it is a systemic disease, involving a wide range of organs and glands.

Also, in certain persons weak adrenal glands may play a role in undermining thyroid function. In fact, in the case of inflammatory disorders of the thyroid, such as Hashimoto's thyroiditis, Grave's disease, and hyperthyroidism, the primary defect is largely adrenal. As well, such diseases are associated with infections of both the adrenals and thyroid, primarily by fungi and even tuberculosis. Ovarian failure may also be connected to the collapse of the thyroid gland.

Ovaries: critical component

This makes it clear that the ovaries, far from an isolated organ system in the lower abdomen, are directly integrated with the entire body. Yet, physicians feel little hesitation of removing them. Can a man imagine what it would be like to have his testicles cut off? They are the ovaries' equals. Removing the testicles should be the absolute last resort. Yet, the surgeon is often cavalier about removing the ovaries. This is despite the fact that this devastates a female's health. It was again Larson who claimed that there is no greater harm done to the female body than the inappropriate removal of the ovaries. He makes it clear that even in the event of known disease every effort should be made only to remove the diseased tissue. Any possible part of the ovary which might be healthy, Larson says, must be salvaged.

When a woman's ovaries are removed, it is highly traumatic. This is an essential organ, which is involved in operations far more complex than mere sexual activity. The ovaries support a woman's entire hormone system. They are needed to help keep this system in balance. They help control metabolism throughout the body, especially in the adrenal and thyroid glands. Thus, when these organs are removed, the entire endocrine system is placed into disarray. Great strain is usually placed on the thyroid gland, and it usually fails.

When even a single ovary is removed, a women's femininity is distorted. Critical functions or aspects, including the inclination for love-making, natural feminine vitality, body conformation, healthy mood/mental state, and normal menstruation, cease or are disrupted. The natural spark, so prominent in vital women, escapes, never to again return. The same consequence occurs in men whose prostate glands are removed or who lose testes. They, too, lose that vital essence, which makes a man so sensual. Yet, through the intake of natural hormones and the proper nutritional supplements, some of this essence can be resurrected. Part of this can be accomplished by boosting sister glands, such as thyroid and adrenals, which compensate for this loss.

The Age Factor

Sluggish thyroid function is a consequence of aging. Virtually everyone suffers a decline in the powers of this gland with time. As described by Mohandas and Gupta in their article *Managing Thyroid Dysfunction in the Elderly* (May 2003) there are certain specific symptoms which are revealing. These include slowing of mental function (poor concentration), poor memory, high cholesterol, intolerance to cold, dryness of the skin, exhaustion, muscular weakness, constipation, poor concentration, and hoarseness. Even deafness can indicate hypothyroidism.

In rare instances the elderly could develop excessive thyroid function, that is hyperthyroidism. This is manifested by rapid heart beat, weight loss, fatigue, nervousness, agitation, tremors, excessive urination, intolerance to heat, and excessive sweating. This most commonly occurs in younger people aged 20 through 45. Usually, elderly people suffer with hypothyroidism. This may be manifested by a modest amount of symptoms: mere tiredness and poor circulation, perhaps with muscular weakness and a degree of sluggish mentation. This why in the elderly the diagnosis of sluggish thyroid syndrome is frequently missed.

The Role of Diet and Nutrition

Diet profoundly influences thyroid function. This gland, while damaged by stress, is even more greatly damaged by a toxic diet. Also, it is readily damaged by specific deficiencies, notably a lack of iodine, amino acids, riboflavin, thiamine, niacin, magnesium, and zinc. Incredibly, a simple deficiency of iodine and amino acids causes extensive damage of this gland. If the deficiency is prolonged or extreme, the gland may undergo atrophy, that is permanent cell death. A deficiency in B vitamins may also result in similar consequences.

In the early 1900s before the role of nutritional deficiency in this organ was firmly established millions of people all over the world suffered from severe thyroid disease. This was in the form of goiter. This is a type of cellular degeneration. The cells over-grow, destroying the infrastructure of the gland. It is all preventable, as well as reversible, strictly through improved nutrition. Iodine is the main deficiency, but, again, there are a wide range of nutrients lacking. Goiter is essentially a gross nutritional deficiency. Also, there is the issue of overall glandular imbalances. So, the most efficient treatment for goiter involves treating the entire endocrine system.

There is another major factor besides deficiency. This is anti-thyroid substances. Incredibly, in nature there are a number of substances, which block iodine absorption. What's more, these substances appear to directly interfere with the action of thyroid hormones. Known as goitrogens, they are found exclusively in vegetation, particularly raw vegetation.

Common vegetables are the major sources of goitrogens. These include primarily vegetables from the mustard family, notably turnips and radishes as well as the cruciferous vegetables, that is Brussels sprouts, cabbage, broccoli, kohlrabi, and cauliflower. Raw carrots and, therefore, carrot juice also contain it. In a thyroid-deficient individual the regular consumption of such vegetables aggravates the condition. In some cases, incredibly, overeating such vegetables may even cause the disorder. In the early 1900s this was well recognized. McCarrison called this "cabbage goiter."

Other sources of goitrogens include raw flaxseed (and, therefore, raw flaxseed oil), raw peanuts, raw almonds, raw walnuts, and raw strawberries. Soy, raw or cooked, is also a major perpetrator. In particular, soy concentrates, such as soy protein, curd, and milk, block thyroid function. This is particularly true for unfermented sources, which retain the full strength of the toxins.

Now that soy is genetically engineered its toxicity is increased. No one should eat commercial soy products. This is particularly true of people with thyroid disorders, who should avoid all commercial soy foods like the plague. Thyroid types must be particularly careful about soy or its derivatives.

People with thyroid disorders must read labels carefully. They should never buy any food which lists soy or its derivatives, especially commercial soy products, which are genetically engineered. GM soy is a deliberate thyroid toxin.

Do not forget, Monsanto and other perpetrators are destroying the rain forests to plant genetically engineered soy. Keep this in mind whenever buying commercial soy products. In fact, anyone who buys 'popular' soy products, such as soy milk and soy-based protein powders, is contributing to the destruction of the rain forest. Regardless, a person would be better off, hormonally, drinking real whole milk instead of consuming such artificial foods. Yet, also for ideal adrenal function the intake of soy milk must be banned. Instead, organic milk, goat's milk, and, if necessary, nut milk should be consumed. Even so, for all types goitrogen-free real organic whole milk is always the best option.

Goitrogens are metabolic inhibitors. Such substances are cyanogenic glycosides, which are a kind of biological form of cyanide. Any chemist knows that cyanide is a metabolic poison. This is why such substances can be so dangerous to the thyroid gland, since it has the highest metabolic rate in the body and is, therefore, highly sensitive to these poisons.

Consider a person living in central or eastern Europe, eating little or no fish and using little if any salt. Then, such a person eats large amounts of traditional foods. These foods include raw cabbage, sauerkraut, Brussels sprouts, raw carrots, cauliflower, radishes, and turnips. As a result, the person becomes lethargic and depressed, even hostile. The throat and neck swells. This is cabbage goiter. Cabbage and similar cruciferous vegetables are commonly consumed in central and eastern Europe. No wonder sluggish thyroid syndrome is a plague in this region.

A high-grain diet is also destructive to the thyroid. This is largely because the thyroid gland is dependent upon salt-bearing foods. Grains contain virtually none of these salts. What's more, grains are devoid of iodine, whereas meats, fish, milk, cheese, and eggs, all of which are salt-bearing, are also relatively iodine-rich. This is particularly true of such animal foods derived from lands rich in iodine such as cattle grazing in Florida, North and South Carolina, Virginia, New Jersey, New York, Ireland/England, and similar iodine-rich regions. Regardless, animal foods are far more dense in iodine than vegetation, the exception, of course, being sea vegetables.

The strict exclusion of animal foods ultimately leads to thyroid decay, that is unless the diet is regularly supplemented with sea vegetation. Yet, incredibly, there are additional substances in animal foods besides the iodine. These are the tissue salts, which are direly needed by the thyroid. Such salts fuel this gland. These is also carnitine in animal foods, which is needed for fuel creation in this gland. Thus, the ideal nutritional support for this organ would include perhaps a combination of iodine-rich vegetation, such as low-pollution kelp/seaweed, and animal sources such as fresh beef, lamb, eggs, and whole milk. Regarding eggs their content of iodine is directly related to the content of the feed. If the feed is lacking, the eggs will fail to be a productive source.

Elimination of animal-source foods leads to a corresponding elimination of food salts, including iodine. It also leads to a drop in the intake of hormones, which are concentrated mainly in animal flesh. This may cause a disruption in endocrine health, as demonstrated by the following case history:

> Ms. T. saw me because of a total decline in her health. She is a vegetarian for religious reasons. She does eat some eggs and cheese. However, because of concerns of allergic intolerance, she recently stopped these. Her health continued to decline. She complained of having no energy, plus her digestion is always disturbed. She is some 30 pounds overweight. A body analysis revealed that she was mainly an adrenal type with a significant thyroid component. Regarding the latter the thickness of her facial skin was revealing: evidence of lymphedema due to low intracellular metabolism. This revealed she has significant hypothyroidism. However, she was not just tired in the morning, which is the thyroid pattern: she was also tired all day long, which is the adrenal pattern.

Treating her as mainly a thyroid type would be an error, resulting in further health problems. Thus, she is not a candidate for thyroid hormone. Rather, a program for boosting, that is normalizing, her thyroid is in order. She was placed on a wild kelp/herbal supplement plus a diet rich in seafood and fish. She was also given undiluted 3x royal jelly capsules, combined with rosemary and sage. The dietary changes were the inclusion of fatty fish, seafood, lamb, and whole goat's milk. She was also instructed to cut back on grains. This was a dramatic change in her diet. Yet, the results were equally dramatic—increased energy, improvement in facial texture, and the loss of over 20 pounds.

The visual signs of hypothyroidism are easy to learn (Note: the thyroid type is based on hypothyroidism). The typical thyroid type is demonstrated in Figures 1 & 2. This is the usual 'look,' which is apple-shaped. However, there are certain variations of this (See Figure 3). Thus a written test, along with the diagram(s), is the best means to determine the type. Blood tests may also be of value. However, these tests usually only reveal the extremes. Incredibly, up to 70% of thyroid function must be lost before blood tests demonstrate the illness. Thus, symptom analysis, combined with body typing, is the most accurate and dependable means to make the diagnosis. Now, thyroid disorders can be determined early, before serious disease results.

Millions of individuals suffer from mild to moderate thyroid dysfunction, but most of them are unaware of it. It is a smoldering disorder that escapes diagnosis. This is known as the Sluggish Thyroid Syndrome. It is perhaps the most commonly occurring hormonal disturbance in America today. Adult women are the primary victims. This sluggishness can ultimately lead to weight gain. Then, by boosting thyroid function this can be reversed, as demonstrated by the following case history:

> Ms. B. has severe hormonal disorders, including thyroid, adrenal, and pituitary imbalances. This caused her to become exceedingly heavy, weighing some 700 pounds. However, her primary type is thyroid. She was placed on large doses of a complex of crude remote-source northern Pacific kelp plus tyrosine and wild oregano, along with wild oregano/Rhus coriaria capsules and undiluted 3x royal jelly. She was also given a formula for supporting ovarian function consisting of spice extracts of fennel, sage, and fenugreek, along with northern Pacific kelp. She took these supplements persistently. As a result, within four months she lost 120 pounds.

As many as one in four Americans suffer from reduced thyroid function. Low body temperature is perhaps the most common consequence of impaired thyroid function. The individual who wears extra layers of clothes, wears socks to bed, or who has "ice cold hands" is typically thyroid deficient. This lowered body temperature affects several critical functions, including digestive enzyme synthesis, stomach acid production, fuel combustion, fat and protein synthesis, white blood cell synthesis/activity, and blood flow. The thyroid gland is also a critical player in the synthesis and activity of sex hormones, so, usually, in hypofunction the blood levels of these hormones are low.

In this syndrome immunity is compromised. This is largely because of the reduced enzyme activity. It is also because of the reduction in body temperature. The immune system operates best at the normal temperature of 98.6 degrees Fahrenheit or higher. When the body is constantly in a low temperature, immune activity is sluggish. Notes R. Mitchell, M.D., of Amarillo, Texas, this increases the vulnerability for opportunistic infections, particularly fungal infections. In fact, one of the cardinal features of a sluggish thyroid is persistent fungal infections of the skin, scalp, and nails. Also, persistent psoriasis and/or eczema is often a signal of sluggish thyroid. As well, the fungus readily populates the deeper tissues, including the internal organs, blood, and bone marrow. The low body core temperature greatly increases the risks for fungal infections. Actually, the majority of people with toenail fungus are the thyroid type.

Psoriasis and eczema are related to germ overgrowth. One reason for this is low oxygen levels in the tissues, which is typical of depressed thyroid function. This leads to the overgrowth of pathogens, such as fungi, strep, and staph, therefore causing the skin lesions.

To determine thyroid status take the following test. A similar test is also found on the internet through Nutritiontest.com. Use such tests, plus the diagrams and signs listed in this book, to determine your status.

Blood tests may also be taken. The combination of the written tests plus blood tests is a good idea. However, for simplicity most people can determine their status through the information found in this book. A score in the moderate category or greater indicates that the person is primarily a thyroid type. Pituitary types usually score high on this test and may even fall in the severe or extreme categories, since with dysfunction of this gland there is always a thyroid component.

Which of these apply to you (each response worth one point, unless otherwise indicated)?

1. fatigue or tiredness
2. tired in the morning and energetic at night (2 points)
3. dry or coarse hair and/or skin
4. slow or slurred speech (2 points)
5. swelling of the face and/or eyelids (2 points)
6. cold hands and feet
7. bloating and indigestion after eating
8. hair loss from the outer third of the eyebrows (3 points)
9. short-term memory loss
10. white spots on the fingernails
11. chronic weight problems
12. easily constipated
13. PMS and/or other menstrual difficulties
14. infertility
15. swelling/puffiness of hands and/or ankles
16. chronic headaches, especially after age forty (2 points)
17. gain weight easily
18. brittle nails or nails which grow slowly
19. bags under eyes
20. mental confusion
21. low motivation
22. hair loss from scalp, especially in women (3 points)
23. easily exhausted
24. heart palpitations
25. drink fluoridated and/or chlorinated water or use fluoridated toothpastes/rinses
26. index finger is considerably shorter than the ring finger on both hands (3 points)
27 joint stiffness
28. require prolonged periods to get "warmed up" after

exposure to cold (2 points)
29. lack of sexual desire
30. slow growing hair and/or nails
31. light or heavy menstrual flow
32. brittle hair
33. cholesterol deposits on the face or eyelids
34. enlarged facial pores
35. poor hand-to-eye coordination
36. hoarseness or coarse voice (2 points)
37. inability to translate thoughts into action
38. become depressed in the winter
39. don't feel like getting up in the morning (2 points)
40. history of ovarian cysts
41. lived in the Great Lakes region for over ten years—
    Illinois, Wisconsin, Indiana, Michigan, Ohio or in
    Canada, Manitoba, Saskatchewan, and Ontario (2 points)
42. high cholesterol level (2 points)
43. low body temperature (2 points)
44. toenail or fingernail fungal infections
45. skin fungal infections
46. psoriasis or eczema
47. head is square or rectangular in shape (2 points)
48. cellulite, especially along the outer thighs
49. sleep until noon (3 points)
50. lack of moons (light colored semicircles) on the index,
    middle, and ring fingers (2 points)
51. history of heart disease, high blood pressure, mitral
    valve prolapse, or atrial fibrillation (2 points)
52. thick multiple vertical ridges on the nails
53. deep horizontal ridges on the nails

54. congestive heart failure
55. muscular weakness
56. sluggish digestion
57. poor circulation
58. furrows on the brow
59. follicular hyperkeratosis (enlarged pores or bumps on back of upper arms)

Your score_____

Any score above 5 is a sign of impaired thyroid function. A score above 10 tells of significant thyroid impairment, while a score above 15 reveals major thyroid impairment. A score of 21 and above represents extreme impairment. At the level of 27 and above the dysfunction is profound. A score above 35 indicates potentially life-threatening dysfunction. Levels above 20 often indicate a coinciding pituitary and/or gonadal component.

The climate factor: another look

Climate plays a crucial role in endocrine function. In general in hot climates the brunt of the stress is on the adrenal glands, while in cold climates the greatest stress is endured by the thyroid. Thyroid types tend to thrive in warm climates. For adrenal types a moderate climate is ideal. Pituitary types also generally do poor in hot climates. This is because of their impaired adrenal status. However, the sunshine in these climates is helpful for all hormonal types.

The pituitary is stressed by both extremes. For adrenal types there is a caution against excess heat and humidity. Intense heat places a great demand on the adrenal glands. Temperate climates, in fact, aid endocrine function, and, thus, moderate climates are ideal for adrenal health. In contrast, humidity creates adrenal stress as well as stress on the pituitary.

The body's ability to deal with climate can be enhanced. This may prove life-saving. Extremes in temperature can cause illnesses, even death. In particular, heat stroke is an issue. Yet, even this is largely preventable. The way to prevent it is to enhance glandular function, especially adrenal and pituitary status. The adrenal glands are directly involved in heat regulation. They are responsible for preventing the retention of excess heat in the body. The adrenal glands control fluid balance, and it is the body fluids, the blood and cellular fluids, which are the body's coolant system. These glands also control salt metabolism. It is salt which acts as the main electrolyte in the blood. The purpose of the salt, as sodium and chloride, is to hold fluid within the blood vessels. If the salt content of the blood drops, so does the fluid level. In the body salt holds and releases heat, just like it does in the oceans.

Salt keeps the blood volume high. Again, it is the blood fluids which are the body's coolant system. Much like in a car radiator, if fluid levels drop precipitously, overheating of the 'engine' occurs. Thus, it is critical to maintain sufficient sodium and chloride levels in the blood. The adrenal glands perform this function. They secrete a special hormone, aldosterone, which prevents salt loss. If the glands are weak, they fail to make sufficient aldosterone, and, therefore, salt levels drop. This decline in salt content is a major cause of overheating, and, thus, during extreme summer weather the result is heat exhaustion or heat stroke. Thus, by strengthening these glands, and, therefore, boosting aldosterone synthesis heat-related illnesses can be prevented.

Salty snacks are of value, that is if they are healthy; for instance, salted nuts, olives, pickles, salted roast beef, unsweetened beef, bison, or turkey jerky (see Americanwildfoods.com), and similar snacks. Pantothenic acid is also a critical factor. This vitamin is the key one for boosting adrenal hormone synthesis. Note: meat and eggs are a top source of this vitamin.

Royal jelly, which provides the needed steroids, also combats heat-related illnesses. Natural-source vitamin C is also needed for steroid synthesis. The best source of such vitamin C is a combination of wild camu camu, acerola, and rose hips. Another source is wild camu camu drops with wild passion fruit. Thus, a combination of these nutrients— wild-source vitamin C plus undiluted royal jelly—is ideal as prevention as well as treatment. A high-grade royal jelly supplement containing adrenal-supporting herbs, such as wild sage and rosemary, is a powerful preventive. A natural vitamin C source such as the aforementioned acerola and/or camu camu should be taken. In fact, I have successfully used this in the treatment of heat stroke, as is represented by the following case history:

> While on a tour in the Sahara I was with a group of medical doctors. One of the attendees, a blond fair-complected woman of northern European descent, who was highly sensitive to sunlight and/or heat, began overheating in the desert sun. Suddenly, she became nauseated and flushed, which are potential signs of heat

stroke. Rapidly, she began to fall into shock. Instead of giving her merely water I gave a salty snack. This was dry roasted salted almonds (pure water would likely accelerate the shock). Plus, I gave her four capsules of undiluted 3x royal jelly combined with pantothenic acid and acerola. While she was obviously declining rapidly, all was stopped and the apparent heat stroke was aborted: all through natural non-toxic therapies.

This is a dramatic real-life example for those who are skeptical. In nature almighty God has created a wide range of cures, whether pharmaceutical companies like it or not. These companies fight the natural option, because it erodes their profits.

The supporters of pharmaceutical companies even spread lies about natural substances, if it serves their purposes. The companies have entire divisions whose purpose is to spread lies about natural substances. By doing so they create doubts in peoples' minds about the safety, as well as power, of natural cures. This is disastrous, because it causes people in need to neglect the pursuit of these cures. As a result, disease is perpetuated, and as demonstrated by the aforementioned case history people even die. These deaths are to a degree the responsibility of the pharmaceutical groups, which discourage the human race from using the God-given gifts. Thus, such groups commit great crimes against humanity as well as against the divine Being.

In cold climates there are also special requirements. The thyroid gland may need to be bolstered. This is proven by the typical native cold-weather diet. Natives eat iodine-rich food, and this nutrient is critical for thyroid strength. They also eat foods rich in vitamins A and D, both of which strengthen this gland. Vitamin A is rapidly used by the cold weather-stressed thyroid. It is also direly needed by the adrenal glands, and the latter are the ones which are also needed to fight cold weather stress. This explains the purpose behind the naturally occurring vitamin A sources in wintery climates, which are fatty fish, organ meats, eggs, butter, cheese, and milk. After all, it is primarily animal foods which are available fresh in the winter. What's more, such foods are the only source for vitamin A. This animal type of vitamin A is the type most readily used by the body. The other type, vegetable vitamin A in the form of beta carotene, is poorly used by the body, especially for thyroid types. Even so, interestingly, beta carotene-rich squash and pumpkins are also winter food. Yet, thyroid types need a good amount of animal-source vitamin A, since they lack the enzyme to efficiently convert the vegetable source to its active forms. Or, the activity of this enzyme is sluggish. This is why thyroid types who adopt a mainly vegetable-based diet quickly develop vitamin A deficiency. This may be manifested by follicular hyperkeratosis, which is enlarged pores on the back of the upper arms as well as light sensitivity at night.

Nutrients needed to strengthen the thyroid's cold-fighting powers include amino acids, vitamin C, vitamin A, vitamin D, zinc, copper, pyridoxine, riboflavin, and iodine. Foods that are ideal for combating cold include fatty fish, organ meats, red meat, poultry (with the skin on), nuts, seeds, nut/seed butters, eggs, whole milk, cheese, and butter. The best supplemental source of natural vitamin A and D is polar-source wild sockeye salmon oil, with naturally occurring astaxanthin. This is the only truly whole food source of high dose vitamins A and D available. The natural astaxanthin prevents this polar empowered salmon oil from becoming rancid. All other sources, including cod liver oil, are heavily refined.

Eating for climate

For metabolic typing adjustments in the diet may be necessary, depending upon the climate. The following are some general recommendations for diet in specific climates:

Hot climate

Seafood and low-fat fish should be emphasized. Fatty fish must be consumed only occasionally. Spices should be used in all dishes, because these help dissipate heat. Fatty meat must be consumed in moderation. Emphasis should be on local fruit and hot desert vegetables such as squash and cucumber. Yogurt is also an excellent food for this climate and is very cooling, especially if consumed with added salt. Raw honey is also a good hot climate food. Salt consumption should be heavy. Fresh greens and local-climate vegetables should be emphasized. Nut and seed consumption should be low. This may be why as a rule fatty nut trees and seed plants do not grow in the tropics. Instead, in the tropics starchy-type foods are found such as peanuts, cashews, cassava, tapioca, and Brazil nuts.

Temperate climate

Seafood and low-fat fish should be consumed instead of fatty fish. However, fatty fish can be consumed in moderation. Fatty meat may also be consumed in moderation, especially lamb and goat. Poultry is ideal. Vegetables and fruit of the local climate should be emphasized. Sea salt consumption is moderate. In moderation fatty nuts and seeds can be consumed. Tropical and sub-tropical fruit should be a major part of the diet, along with light fish and seafood.

Cold climate

Here, the intake of fat should be high. This is crucial for efficiently thriving in such a climate. Regarding ocean species only cold water fish and deep sea seafood, such as wild salmon, halibut, mackerel, lobster, and crab, should be eaten. Low-fat fish consumption should be limited if any. The emphasis should be on the fatty fish, since the fish oils and fat soluble vitamins are essential for combating cold weather stress. For instance, a polar or grizzly bear would reject low-fat fish. It must have the fats to survive. In order to gain optimal health follow nature. Organic red meat is also recommended, as is local game. For starches whole potatoes with skins and wild rice are acceptable. Brown rice should be eaten in moderation and ideally be cut 50/50 with wild rice. Nut and seed consumption should be liberal. Sea salt consumption is moderately high to high.

The adrenal type (medium-to-fast metabolizer)

The adrenal type is often a combination of several types. Usually, such types suffer from overall endocrine imbalances. Yet, the major glandular system of concern is the adrenals. In this section the attempt will be to determine if the adrenal component is the dominant one. Tens of millions of people living in the Western world suffer from primary adrenal disorders. This is largely due to the consumption of processed and adulterated foods.

It is also related to inheritance, that is if the parents were consumers of such foods. Children born to parents who were/are sugar addicts often develop this type, especially if they, too, are big consumers. The condition may also be related to alcohol consumption. This is in the event that either the mother or father—or both—were regular drinkers. Also, children allowed to drink at a young age are likely to develop it. Teenage drinkers, especially those who develop sudden addictions, are likely of the adrenal metabolic type.

The standard Western diet is destructive. The brunt of the damage is suffered by the glandular system, with the adrenals suffering perhaps the most significant damage. Anyone brought up on a modern or Western diet is vulnerable for the development of adrenal collapse.

In this metabolic type there is usually a history of physical weakness. This is the person who is always exhausted. Often, the individual overcomes this through will power and, perhaps, exercise. Yet, there is an inherent tendency towards weakness and vulnerability.

The reason for the weakness is easily explained. Steroid hormones are essential for muscular strength. The muscles and bones are nourished by these hormones.

Adrenal types are often very gentle. Some adrenal types are delicate and loving. They are also very sensitive. Adrenal types are often highly instinctive. They may also be intuitive. With a tendency to worry excessively they can become somewhat paranoid. However, they can use such senses to their advantage, for instance, for clairvoyance, financial endeavors, inventions, and similar productive pursuits. Even so, there are certain derogatory aspects to this sensitivity.

Often, concentration is greatly impaired. This is the person who finds it difficult to focus on anything. There may be a sensation of internal nervousness, even anxiety. Depression is common, as is insomnia. However, nervousness and agitation are more common than the former. Even so, in some cases there may be the opposite consequence, that is there may be a kind of mental dullness and confusion.

Joseph Tintera, M.D., one of the world's finest endocrinologists, was one of the first to discover the connection of the mind with weak adrenals. Incredibly, in his respected list of the top nine symptoms of weak adrenals six of them are 'mental.' These symptoms are poor concentration, apprehension, nervousness, irritability, depression, and insomnia.

Typically, in this type there are certain physical characteristics, which are revealing. The individual often has a long index finger versus the ring—normal is when the index finger is longer the ring finger. Or, the fingers may be the same length, which is also indicative of the adrenal type. The face is usually thin or at least thinner than the thyroid types. Puffiness is rare. Often, the facial bones of the chin are smaller than normal. Typically, there is a receding chin. Also, the facial bones may be smaller than normal. The roof of the mouth is usually small and arched. The eyes are often sunken, and there may be dark circles under the eyes. The hair is medium fine to fine. In men, usually, the hair on the head is thinner than normal, and there may be male-pattern baldness, although this also is common in thyroid types. Additionally, there is a tendency for the hair to be straight rather than curly. It may be wispy. In a blond and blue-eyed person fine straight hair is virtual proof of this type.

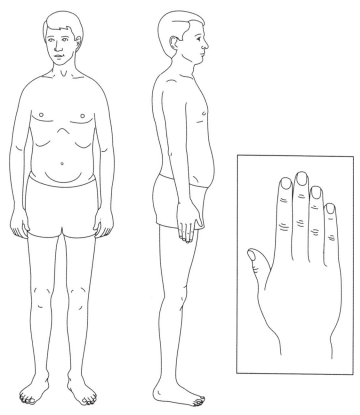

FIG. 4 Male adrenal body type

In the pure adrenal type the metabolic rate is generally rapid. Yet, such adrenal types tend to be thin. If they are heavy, they usually have a thyroid and/or pituitary component. For adrenal types weakness is the predominant symptom. Also, typically, the adrenal types are unable to cope with stress. They are often worriers, unable to ever have settled minds. They often appear unhappy, largely because they are constantly worrying or, perhaps, fuming about their health.

Adrenal types can be overweight. However, they are usually slender. According to the book *Organotherapy* published in the 1920s by C. W. Carrick Co. the main symptoms are fatigue, a feeling of being "run-down," sensitivity to cold and/or cold extremities, low blood pressure, weak heart pulse, irregular heart beat, sluggish metabolism, constipation, sluggish digestion, reduced blood count, and mental exhaustion or depression. Now it is known that there are virtually hundreds of symptoms of this

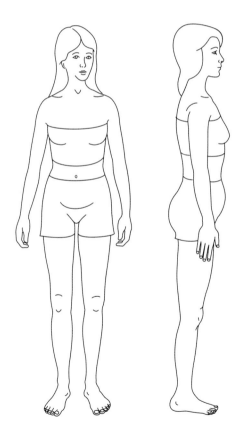

FIG. 5 Female adrenal body type

condition. The adrenal glands control both physical and mental functions. In addition to these mainly physical symptoms there are also mental symptoms such as panic attacks, anxiety, compulsive behavior, agitation, and temper tantrums. Thus, it is no surprise that adrenal problems are often confused with a host of other diseases, including psychological conditions. This leads to an incorrect diagnosis as well as the prescription of unnecessary, in fact, dangerous medications. Millions of Americans have been hospitalized and even institutionalized under the diagnoses of mental diseases when, actually, the entire problem was adrenal weakness.

The true adrenal type is a sort of weakling. These individuals are always in need of help. Their will power may be strong. However, their body fails to follow this. They are the people who have difficulty opening up a stuck car door or removing a tight jar lid. They are the types who are easily drained by stress. A mere emotional reaction can devastate them. If tremendous pressure is placed upon them, they collapse, sleeping to recover. This is far from a psychological issue, rather, it is strictly physical, that is the diminished ability to cope due to weakened adrenal function. Another type is tall and lanky but not necessarily weak. This type has a relatively fast metabolism, and so even when eating large quantities of food rarely gains excessive weight. However, if weight is gained, it is usually in the buttocks or hips or around the lower abdomen.

The adrenal type often develops bizarre symptoms. Usually, doctors are unable to understand these symptoms. Yet, the symptoms are real and often devastating. It is the adrenal individual who looks relatively healthy, that is who has no overt signs of disease, but inside feels generally "lousy." Such a person complains constantly of a wide range of seemingly vague symptoms, including digestive problems, heartburn, aches, various back pains, especially in the upper mid- to lower-back, headaches, nervousness, dizziness, fatigue, and weakness. Adrenal types tend to be over-workers, and often they are compulsive. Usually, they crave salt as well as sugar. They can easily become sugar addicts. Or, they may alternate sugar binges with binges of eating salty snacks. They are the typical persons who must have salty snacks. They may also crave alcohol and occasionally over-indulge in it. However, alcohol usually makes them sick, so that they avoid it.

Lack of a strong voice is typical of the adrenal type. Often, a person must strain to hear them. They may even have a dragging voice, which is tiresome and/or monotonous. They may be whiners, who seem to never stop complaining or nagging. Frequently, they talk endlessly, and no one can speak even a word between. They may give the appearance of being nervous, even agitated or upset. Such individuals often exhibit aggravating habits such as being fidgety or repetitive tapping of the feet. The shopkeeper who is unable to stop talking is typically hypoadrenal. Thus, their hyperactivity is a mere compensation, a sign of adrenal weakness. These people have very little coping capacity. In contrast, truly calm people who can easily cope usually have strong adrenal glands.

Even so, again, adrenal types may also be the silent type, saying little. Some adrenal people are quiet and may even be the opposite of the nervous type, virtually tongue-tied. The adrenal behavior depends to a large degree upon the personality. With this condition the quiet type is equally as common as the talkative bore. In fact, shyness is a common symptom of adrenal weakness. This is, perhaps, even more common than nervousness. This shyness, even physical weakness, is why people with this type are often taken advantage of.

The adrenal glands are the primary organ system for fighting stress. They are responsible for warding off the ill effects of every conceivable mental and/or physical stressor. Emotional strain causes a significant disruption of adrenal function. Anger is perhaps the most devastating of all mental stressors. Researchers have discovered that its negative effects on adrenal function are profound. In people with adrenal weakness anger greatly devastates their systems. They must strive to remain calm. Otherwise, they will destroy themselves. With worry and fretting people with adrenal insufficiency think their way into adrenal failure. Thus, it is essential that they remain calm and worry-free.

Because the adrenal type is physically weak, he/she may be the subject of torment when growing up. Even later in life, if joining with the wrong person, this type may be tormented. The fact is the adrenal type is regarded by others as weak, that is physically, and so unable to defend himself/herself. Yet, actually, adrenal types are often capable of defending themselves. However, they only do so in life-threatening circumstances. What's more, they are rarely if ever bullies. Rather, they are the ones who are bullied.

This type is also typically fine-boned. Although they are often relatively slender, occasionally, they are obese.

Many adrenal types have a refined, almost sophisticated, appearance. They are usually delicate, physically and emotionally. They are highly sensitive and react excessively to stimuli. These are the types that are sensitive to every kind of noise, smell, and sensation, even people's auras, that is energy fields. This sensitivity, however, can be of value, especially in the business world or in other human interactions. The adrenal type may sense critical issues, even potential traumatic events, thereby preventing disaster. This sensitive type is the ideal one to have in the room when interviewing candidates. Such a type will sense issues which will be undetected by the thyroid or muscular types.

For the adrenal type the sensitivity to smells is well published. It may be 1,000 and up to 100,000 times greater than normal. This acute sensitivity returns to normal once the function of the gland is revived.

Diet has an enormous impact upon adrenal function. There are many foods or substances in the American diet which damage these glands. In particular, refined sugar is a major adrenal toxin. It stresses the function of these glands more so than any other food. The adrenals can well handle fats, that is the natural types, and protein, but they must work enormously to process sugar. Truly, the adrenals are unable to process refined sugar, not without undergoing self-destruction. Every time it is consumed a portion of the adrenals is destroyed. This is especially true of refined sugar, which is an absolute adrenal poison. If a person consumes it to the excess, the glands are severely stressed. The glands must pump out steroid hormones, millions of molecules at a time, to deal with it. Sugar causes a depletion from the glands of its hormones.

In contrast, protein and natural fats never cause this depletion. The exception is allergy. This is because it is the adrenals which must process allergic reactions. Thus, if a person is allergic to a fatty food, for instance, butter, the adrenals must deal with it, and therefore, depletion of adrenal steroids may occur. Or, if a person is allergic to shrimp, which is mostly protein, this can cause an intense allergic reaction, which consumes adrenal hormones. Yet, this is nothing compared to the damage caused by noxious sugar.

For the vast majority of the population it is sugar and sugar alone which causes adrenal depletion. The point is when refined sugar is consumed, the adrenal glands are forced to deal with it. This is because adrenal steroids are needed to balance blood sugar. The sugar is greatly depleting steroid levels, causing vast physiological disruption. As the glands lose an increasingly large amount of steroid hormones blood sugar is impossible to properly balance. The person becomes dependent upon sugar for survival. If the sugar consumption is continuous, these glands are drained of all vitality.

Of course, the sugar consumption usually continues unabated. This is when the cell destruction occurs. Sugar even causes internal bleeding within this organ. Researchers have proven this by examining the adrenal glands during surgery. They have also found that when the glands are damaged by either trauma or poor diet, they may readily become infected, notably by *Mycobacterium tuberculosis* and fungi. So, it is not just the sugar, it is what the sugar does to the tissues that is the issue.

As a result of repeated sugar consumption the adrenal glands lose their important stores of adrenal steroids. The vitamin-mineral content of these glands also declines, since sugar aggressively depletes these nutrients. It is a refined food, and the body doesn't know what to do with it. So, this stress is borne by the adrenals.

This refined poison, this adulterated, bleached, and nutrient-free 'sweetener,' devastates adrenal function. These glands must compensate greatly merely to prevent tissue collapse. As a result, the glands become swollen and inflamed. In the extreme internal bleeding develops, ultimately resulting in cell death. This has devastating consequences upon health. Here, too, is when various germs set in, causing chronic infection of the already diseased gland.

Ultimately, if the sugar consumption is unabated, the glands atrophy, that is die. Medically, this is known as necrosis. It is a kind of internal gangrene. This is when the glands are readily infected, all largely a consequence of the excessive consumption of refined sugar. At this point the individual's health declines massively. He/she usually becomes a fulminant sugar addict, since virtually all adrenal reserve is lost, and thus, the sugar is consumed to maintain an artificial level of blood glucose. With the loss of this reserve there is no means to keep the blood sugar balanced. Thus, the person becomes dependent upon artificially raising blood sugar, therefore explaining the continuous intake of this poison. In fact, here the addiction is complete, and this is very difficult to break. In many ways this is worse than cocaine addiction.

Attempting to control such individuals is virtually impossible. Attempting to take the sugar away from them is like fighting a war, the battle usually being won by the sugar addict. In the normal case when sugar is eaten, the adrenal glands, difficult for them as it is, would eventually stabilize the blood sugar. As a result of persistent sugar intake, when the adrenal glands become weak or depleted, this becomes impossible. The blood sugar ultimately falls, the sugar cravings become uncontrollable, and the individual succumbs to his sweet devices. This is a highly destructive sequence, which ultimately leads to physical and mental collapse, in fact, the individual's destruction.

Some adrenal types can survive on fat and protein alone. The best proteins are from animal foods. The fat should ideally be virtually saturated. Adrenal types thrive on such fat, although they may not need them in huge quantities. The best vegetable oils are those high in saturates such as wild red palm oil, extra virgin coconut oil, and extra virgin olive oil.

Yet, while such individuals may initially gain strength from such a diet, with time, the diet becomes monotonous and counterproductive. In moderation, complex carbohydrates must be added. Vegetables are less desirable, because they are exceedingly high in potassium. This distorts the sodium to potassium ratio. This creates great stress on the adrenal glands by depleting the sodium-preserving hormone known as aldosterone. Large amounts of vegetables may even poison these glands. Fruit is superior. In general, the following fruit should be consumed due to their low sugar content. Such fruit include melons, berries, papaya, kiwi, strawberries, lemons, limes, sour oranges, and grapefruit. The citrus fruit and melons should be sprinkled with sea salt. Cooked fruit or fruit juice should be minimized or avoided. The cooking increases the sugar content through a process known as caramelization. Yet, again, if cooked fruit is consumed, salt should be added. Even so, in some cases fruit of any type may be poorly tolerated. Here, the diet should be primarily meat, seafood, and salads, with perhaps organic eggs and whole milk products. This will rest the adrenal glands, until starches and sugars can be safely added.

In most cases the adrenal type can handle a good amount of cooked starch. The best types are the unprocessed or complete starches. These include wild and brown rice, brown rice crackers, baked potato with the skin, rice polish/bran (especially in the form of a combined powder with crushed flaxseed and red sour grape), oat bran, and baked squash. Such starches blend well with salt, the latter being greatly needed by the adrenals. Baked sweet potatoes are often poorly tolerated, but raw is fine. Raw honey may be tolerated, since it is a kind of medicine. Syrup of yacon root, an Andean product, is beneficial. The latter has virtually a zero glycemic index and is best when combined with cinnamon extract. This is the ideal sweetener for people with weak adrenals. Coarse, whole grains may also be tolerated. Raw maca extract is powerful.

In some instances honey is poorly tolerated, especially in adrenal types who also have fungal infections and/or severe blood sugar disorders. If the fungus is eliminated, the honey will be more readily tolerated. Or, as an alternative the remote-source, raw, low-glycemic yacon root extract may be used. This is in the form of a syrup, which has a wonderful sweet/caramel taste.

Multiple spice extract normalizes blood sugar. Such an extract consists of concentrates of wild myrtle, plus cumin, cinnamon, fenugreek, and wild oregano. Available as the premium, wild, hand-picked type, this has been researched at Georgetown University, Washington, D.C., and found to dramatically reduce blood sugar. In animals reared as diabetics as reported in the journal *Molecules and Chemistry*, 2001, a near 50% reduction in blood sugar levels was achieved in only one dose.

This multiple spice extract is a potent means to regulate the blood sugar. Thus, when taking it, tasty and healthy carbohydrate-rich foods, such as baked potatoes, brown rice, and honey, are better tolerated. This means the multiple spice extract has a hormone-like action, driving sugars into cells, so they can be burned as energy. This effect also includes an improvement in the digestion of carbohydrates, as well as sugars. A final effect of this complex is rather dramatic. This is because such a multiple spice extract greatly curbs sugar cravings. So, this specific complex can dramatically eliminate sugar addiction. For sugar addiction simply take a capsule or more with every meal. Warning: this complex may increase the appetite for healthy, powerful foods such as natural meats, fish, vegetables, and fruit. However, it does not cause weight gain, but rather, it induces weight loss. Such a multiple spice complex is useful for reducing starch cravings.

Adrenal types are often sugar addicts. This is the typical extreme addict, who is exceptionally difficult to cure. This difficulty can be modified by the use of multiple spice extracts, yacon syrup, and concentrates of royal jelly. Also, the sugar addiction may be a symptom of a more dire underlying problem. This is the dilemma of chronic fungal or yeast infection. The fungi and yeasts cause ravenous cravings for sugar, which are virtually impossible to control.

So, what can be done? How can such fulminant addicts be helped? Again, the adrenal hormones are lacking, so there is no means for the body to manage blood sugar levels. This explains cravings for sweets. In fact, this is evidence that there is virtually complete depletion of adrenal hormones. The glands, finally poisoned into oblivion, are unable to make enough steroid hormones to combat the crisis. Such intensive damage may be caused by other factors, including drug abuse, prescription drugs, alcohol, persistent psychic stress, and prolonged starvation-type diets. The early symptoms of adrenal failure include fatigue, muscle weakness, insomnia, persistent mid- to lower-back pain, severe or uncontrollable cravings for sugar and/or salt, uncontrollable behavior (in children), mood swings, PMS, agitation, violent tendencies, personality defects, and chronic headaches. This adrenal failure syndrome is the direct result of high sugar consumption. Cocaine also poisons the adrenal glands.

The type of failure seen in cocaine addicts is exceptionally fierce. The only hope for such individuals is to replenish the adrenal steroids. This can be done through a combination of diet and supplements. The diet is simple. It is super-rich in protein, fat, and, yes, cholesterol. It is low in refined sugars and starches. Actually, for adrenal types any kind of refined sugar is taboo. So in most instances are wheat, rye, corn, and beans. Instead, the diet is mainly meat, poultry, fish, eggs, milk products, and fruit, with some vegetables. Certain complex carbohydrates are allowed, for instance, wild rice, rice bran, baked potato, and oat bran. However, all refined sugars and starches must be omitted, as must be corn and wheat. For this type the most ideal vegetables are salad greens. Tomatoes and avocados are preferable to carrots, string beans, cauliflower, and broccoli.

In all these examples aggressive therapy is the answer. True, the blood sugar must be controlled, through the intake of natural complexes, particularly multiple spice extracts. However, in addition the fungi must be purged from the blood for the cravings to be controlled, even eliminated. This again is through the intake of extracts of wild spices. Oil of wild oregano, as well as oil of remote-grown cumin, are potent antifungal agents, which are completely safe for human consumption. Both these substances dramatically curb the cravings for sugar, largely by destroying fungi. Cumin also has a direct action on the pancreas. This action causes insulin to be more readily used by the cells. For medicinal purposes cumin extract, as the steam distilled spice oil, may be found in the multiple spice oil complex, as gelatin capsules and oil in a dropper bottle, or as edible oil of cumin in a base of extra virgin olive oil.

For this metabolic type a purely vegetable-based diet is unacceptable. This is because vegetation has the wrong balance of salts. It is too high in potassium, while excessively low in sodium. Such a mineral ratio causes great stress upon the adrenals, leading to the depletion of the salt-saving hormone aldosterone. In contrast, meat is high in sodium, as well as chloride, while relatively low in potassium. It has the ideal sodium/chloride to potassium ratio. Thus, it fails to weaken adrenal status, rather, strengthens it. Therefore, fresh red meat, the richest source of sodium and chloride salts, is the ideal adrenal-replenishing food. For vegans and vegetarians with adrenal syndrome who follow a no-meat diet it is critical to use sea salt on food liberally, but they should use only the unbleached type. This increased intake of salt will minimize the salt loss, which is inevitable on such diets. Also, such individuals should take wild-source triple salt capsules with each meal (see Appendix A). Plus, celery and celery root are high in sodium.

People with depleted adrenal glands may gain great strength from reasonable quantities of red meat, including organic beef, bison, elk, venison, antelope, and similar foods. These foods give them a fairly prolonged degree of stamina, usually for hours. Poultry and fish are also ideal but not as powerful as red meat. Usually, a 10- to 12-ounce steak gives such person a great sense of strength. This is especially true if it is eaten at night. Many adrenal types must eat red meat as often as possible. They may combine this with complex carbohydrates such as a baked potato or chunks of raw sweet potato.

Red meat contains a critical adrenal component. This is cholesterol. Thus, this food is a complete one for these glands, as it contains the three most critical substances, which replenish it. These are cholesterol, sodium, and chloride. Another option is free-range bison and elk, which while lower in fat are also rich in tissue salts.

Red meat contains another critical factor, known as pantothenic acid. This vitamin is the key one for stimulating cholesterol synthesis. Without it cholesterol production throughout the body declines and, ultimately, stalls. Meat, not vegetation, is by far the best source of this vitamin. However, considerable amounts can also be procured from eggs, whole milk products, poultry, and the brans/germs of whole grains. Vitamin C is also critical for adrenal hormone synthesis. This explains the emphasis on this diet of fruit versus vegetables. Additionally, refined sugar depletes this vitamin. In extreme cases of adrenal weakness it is necessary to supplement the diet with these nutrients.

In certain cases adrenal types don't tolerate excessive amounts of fatty meats. This is true of those with major pituitary weakness. In such types lean red meat, such as grass-fed bison, venison, and elk, may be better tolerated as well as fatty fish and seafood. Regardless, for adrenal types a plant-only diet is a poor choice and usually leads to weakness and exhaustion.

Supplements derived from natural sources are far more regenerative than the synthetic. Natural vitamin C feeds the glands, while the synthetic fails to do so. Crude extracts of certain fruits and herbs offer considerable amounts of natural vitamin C, for instance, capsules containing pure wild Amazon-source camu camu plus extracts of acerola and rose hips. The latter contains over 75 mg of all-natural vitamin C per capsule. That is an incredibly dense supply of this natural vitamin. Plus, in contrast to the commercial types it is non-GMO. This is also available as wild camu camu drops, which is in a raw state, along with wild raw extract of passion fruit.

Pantothenic acid also helps reverse adrenal weakness as well as sugar toxicity. Again, this is found mainly in animal foods, although the brans of grain contain considerable amounts. In the event of sugar- or alcohol-induced adrenal damage it is necessary to rebuild the glands. Use the following protocol to strengthen glands and to prevent them from further damage.

How to correct sugar addiction and adrenal exhaustion

Royal jelly is the ideal source of naturally occurring pantothenic acid. This can be consumed in the form of a stabilized paste or lyophilized powder in a capsule. Thus, in addition to the diet the following food extracts must be taken:

- unprocessed 3x lyophilized royal jelly, ideally combined with wild rosemary and sage; use only the undiluted form
- stabilized paste of raw royal jelly in a crude cold-pressed

pumpkinseed oil base
- crude extract of high vitamin C fruit, consisting of a combination of camu camu, rose hips, and acerola
- crude rice bran/polish extract in a powdered form
- multiple spice extract for eliminating sugar cravings
- juice of wild oregano (natural hydrosol from the hand-picked wild plant)
- crude extract of maca root or roasted maca coffee

The ideal foods for strengthening the adrenal glands are those which are low in potassium but relatively high in sodium and chloride. Also, foods rich in cholesterol greatly strengthen these glands. So do vitamin C-rich foods, although many such foods are also high in potassium.

Foods rich in cholesterol are relatively few. These foods include:

- chicken egg yolks (from free range or organic chickens only)
- quail eggs
- duck or turkey eggs
- fresh organic red meat
- fatty fish
- organic liver or kidney
- organic sweetbreads (thymus)
- free range/organic poultry (always with skin on)
- organic or wild duck
- organic butter
- organic whole milk or cream
- organic or imported cheese
- organic quark
- organic sour cream and yogurt

For vitamin C-rich food select from the following list:

- lemons and limes
- sour oranges and/or blood oranges
- grapefruit
- kiwi
- papaya
- wild berries
- organic strawberries
- organic tomatoes
- organic red sweet peppers (dust with sea salt)

Notice there is only one vegetable on this list. This is because such foods fail to regenerate this gland. This includes vegetable juices, which should largely be avoided. Fruit juices are an exception, as is fresh fruit. Remember, too, that tomatoes are a fruit. So are avocados. Thus, they are acceptable on this plan. Tomatoes are richer in vitamin C than most vegetables. They can act as a 'vegetable' replacement but must be salted liberally.

Fruit supplies much-needed vitamin C, which the adrenals require for hormone synthesis. Plus, it provides organic acids, which also aid in adrenal hormone synthesis. For instance, tomato juice is 'fruit juice' and, thus, is allowed. V-8 is disallowed, as it is mostly a vegetable juice. Carrot juice is unacceptable. However, freshly squeezed orange, blood orange, and grapefruit juice are ideal. So is tangerine juice. In the frozen section of health food stores are fresh frozen citrus juices: these are highly adrenal regenerative. If these are unavailable, opt for the commercial orange and grapefruit juice "not from concentrate" in the milk carton containers. Olives and avocados are two other key fruit which assist in the adrenal repair plan. This is because while these, too, are high in potassium they contain a number of adrenal regenerative factors. Extra virgin olive oil contains saturated fats. The hydrogen molecules of the oil aid in adrenal steroid synthesis. Avocados are the top vegetable or, rather, fruit source of pantothenic acid.

Extra virgin olive oil is an ideal oil for adrenal regeneration. So is crude, dark-colored pumpkinseed oil (Austrian source, fortified). This is because the latter oil is rich in precursors for adrenal steroids known as phytosterols. Crude, cold-pressed remote-source (Turkish) sesame oil may also prove invaluable. Avocado oil is also rich in adrenal-nourishing saturated fats. What's more, avocados, pumpkin seeds, and olives, being rich in fat, help balance blood sugar. By adding sea salt the negative effects of the vegetable potassium is cancelled. Thus, guacamole with plenty of salt is an ideal adrenal food. So are salted olives (the olives are traditionally pickled in brine) and pumpkin seeds.

When on the adrenal diet, be sure to always eat avocados, as well as tomatoes, with added salt. Slice these fruit up, and sprinkle with prodigious amounts of sea salt. Coat with extra virgin olive oil, cold-pressed remote-source sesame oil, and/or crude Austrian pumpkinseed oil (fortified with fennel and rosemary oils).

If eating dark greens, be sure to salt them aggressively. For instance, here is how to make spinach for the adrenal insufficient. Cook it, and drain the water (this eliminates a considerable amount of potassium). Reheat it again in a small amount of water, and discard the juice. Then, add salted butter and extra sea salt. Or, make creamed spinach using real cream (no wheat flour) plus added sea salt. This will convert the spinach from adrenal-toxic to adrenal-nourishing.

For the adrenal type all vegetables should be drizzled with extra virgin olive oil, crude pumpkinseed oil, or wild red palm oil, and/or cooked with butter, even cream. A heavy hand must be used with the salt shaker, using sea salt. Salads should be drizzled heavily with avocado, crude pumpkinseed oil, and/or extra virgin olive oil. Add crumbled organic or imported feta cheese. Top with sliced turkey, beef, or avocado, if desired. This is an ideal food/menu for the adrenal glands.

Remember, carbohydrates, particularly refined types, such as white sugar, rice, and flour, cause the loss of adrenal hormones. Again, so does an excess of potassium-rich foods such as too many vegetables. This is why salad made from fruit—olives, avocado, and tomatoes—is most ideal for adrenal types. Vitamin C regenerates these hormones, so the high vitamin C content of certain fruit cancels any negatives from the sugar. As well, little can replace the adrenal-nourishing power of natural meats, rich in cell-nourishing salts and pantothenic acid.

Meat, as well as milk products and eggs, is rich in riboflavin, yet another substance direly needed by the adrenal glands. This vitamin, which is commonly deficient in the American diet, is needed for oxygen delivery within cells. In the adrenal glands it serves to speed the synthesis of cholesterol; it is an essential part of the step-wise creation of this molecule. Riboflavin keeps the oxygen metabolism within the adrenal glands in ideal condition. Thus, it is crucial for the health of this organ. Without it, oxygen metabolism in these glands is disrupted, which can lead to a decline in adrenal hormone synthesis. In the extreme the lack of riboflavin places the adrenal cells at a high risk. Oxygen can no longer be efficiently metabolized. Toxic forms of oxygen are produced. Steroid hormones can no longer be efficiently synthesized. The result is cell damage and death. Top sources of riboflavin are primarily animal foods, particularly organ meats, red meats, whole milk products, and eggs, although avocados contain lesser but significant amounts. Thus, diets which restrict the aforementioned foods lead to riboflavin deficiency.

Vinegar is concentrated acetic acid. This is precisely the substance needed by the body to make cholesterol. The adrenals, ovaries, testes, and liver all make cholesterol. All do so from acetic acid, known medically as acetate. Thus, by supplying acetate in the form of vinegar steroid synthesis can be boosted. It is a simple equation: supply the body with the raw materials it needs, and let it heal itself. Thus, vinegar can be used extensively on the adrenal gland regenerative diet. Again, vinegar contains the precursor for the synthesis of adrenal, as well as ovarian and testicular, hormones.

Salt is also an adrenal regenerative. The only vegetable which is truly regenerative is kelp. This is largely because while kelp is high in potassium it is even higher in sodium— far higher. Plus, kelp contains dense amounts of iodine, which boosts adrenal hormone synthesis. Chlorella, being low in sodium, is less helpful. However, it is an excellent cleansing agent.

Fishbein claims in his medical encyclopedia that sodium loss is a critical factor in the cause of the typical symptoms of adrenal collapse, which are fatigue, weakness, and other vague symptoms. He states that a high intake of sodium with a low intake of potassium is the crucial formula for medicating these glands. This would imply the need to restrict the intake of high potassium foods, while instead consuming those foods relatively low in this mineral or which at least have the counteracting tissue salts. Again, low-potassium foods include red meat, eggs, cheese, whole milk, yogurt, quark, kefir, butter, poultry, seafood, fish, and organ meats. What's more, all such foods are relatively high in salts.

In the book *Organotherapy* the extreme of adrenal exhaustion is listed as Addison's disease. Today, this is regarded as a rare condition. However, physicians fail to understand all its symptoms and, therefore, do not realize how truly common it is. Addison's is regarded as fatal. In the 1930s, when this condition was well recognized, it wasn't regarded as rare. This was because physicians were familiar with the presentation. Today, highly sick people present to the doctors' offices with either Addison's or, perhaps, pre-Addison's, and it is diagnosed otherwise. What's more, people who die of Addison's-like syndromes are rarely listed as such: the cause of death is disguised under a wide range of other causes. Doctors simply are unaware of the tremendous role played by extreme adrenal exhaustion in the cause of disease. People with adrenal collapse may readily die of lung infections, for instance, pneumonia. They may also die of sudden death from unknown causes. As well, collapsed lung occurs most commonly in people with weak adrenals and may actually be a sign of hidden TB infection.

Such people are exhausted. Their immune systems are weak. Doctors fail to recognize the cause of the exhaustion. This results in overwhelming misery. Plus, it results in deaths, which are preventable.

According to *Organotherapy* Addison's was first discovered in 1855 by Thomas Addison. Interestingly, this is the same time that refined sugar was systematically introduced to the public.

Addison's is described as a disease usually of middle-aged people, striking females more often than males. The full blown variety is rare. What is more common is a low level type, which afflicts countless millions. It occurs gradually and is represented by a kind of overall exhaustion, disinterest, or even apathy. It is the syndrome of aches and pains and a generalized feeling of being ill. The blood pressure is low, and the body temperature is subnormal. There may also be a low red blood count or at least low-normal count, the latter only being discovered by an astute physician.

The reference range will create confusion here. It is a physiological decline, and a reduction in the red cell count to less than ideal is an early warning sign. Full-fledged anemia is more rare but is an obvious sign. The hemoglobin may also be slightly reduced. Also, the total white count may be slightly or even moderately low. This is a sign of not only low adrenal output but also chronic fungal and/or viral infection.

Digestive disturbances are common. This is manifested predominately by vague digestive distress, heartburn, bloating, diarrhea, constipation, and even vomiting. This is in the extreme case. More commonly there is an alternating character to the diarrhea and constipation. Pebble-like stools are common. The individual is often visibly nervous or has nerve-related signs such as tics, twitchings, sweaty palms, sweaty feet, and bizarre movements or tapping of the feet. Joint pain is common, especially in the upper back, mid-lower back, as well as the neck. There is usually constant stiffness of the neck and upper back. Often, sleep is impossible, even though the person is exhausted. There may be sleeping or napping on the job. There may also be difficult arising. The individual who sleeps till noon is typically Addisonian. There is muscular fatigue. The person with this condition might find it difficult to have the discipline for strenuous work. Yet, the most characteristic of all symptoms is the extreme tiredness or weakness, a kind of worn-out effect, often combined with obvious muscular fatigue. Addison claimed that a key in making the diagnosis is to determine if the exhaustion is the main symptom, that is the symptom which has existed since the beginning of the condition.

In a high percentage of true Addison's disease cases there are pigment deposits, which are tell-tale signs. This is next in importance to the extreme weakness, which, by itself, can establish the diagnosis. These spots usually occur after the onset of the weakness. They may develop on any region of the body and may also develop on the mucous membranes. However, they are most commonly found on the face, neck, back of the hands, lips, anal folds, knuckles, and similar surfaces.

It is difficult to diagnose Addison's or any lesser adrenal disorder merely from blood tests. Symptom analysis is ideal, because the degree of damage is always represented by predictable signs and symptoms. Again, this is largely a sugar-induced disease. There was no such disease until refined sugar was introduced. Actually, in 1840 such sugar was made common by the passing out of sugar packets to the population. This was done to cause the people to become addicted to it. Stress is a secondary factor. The combination of a high sugar diet plus stress usually precipitates this disease. Then, too, if, metabolically, a person is an adrenal type the potential is high for its development.

When the adrenals become damaged or infected, this results in an Addison's-like syndrome. For instance, tens of millions of Westerners suffer from defective, damaged, and infected adrenals. Thus, Addison's-like diseases are far more common than is recognized. What's more, there exists a kind of sub-clinical Addison's disease, not enough to be full-blown but, rather, a sort of chronic adrenal dysfunction, which leads to a gradual decline in health. This is a serious condition, and the degree of seriousness varies from a state of constant exhaustion to full-blown life-threatening disease.

The adrenals are vital to life. Moderate to severe damage always compromises the body. The usual result is chronic weakness and/or serious disease. A list of diseases which result from damaged adrenals includes chronic fatigue syndrome, fibromyalgia, lupus, Crohn's disease, tuberculosis, diabetes, heart failure, asthma, viral syndrome, Epstein-Barr infection, leukemia, and systemic fungal infections. Also, numerous skin disorders may result, including hives, eczema, vitiligo, alopecia, and psoriasis. Other conditions which are related to weak or diseased adrenal glands include anxiety disorders, allergies, rhinitis, sinusitis, acne, and bronchitis.

Regardless of the cause, damage to the adrenal glands, including adrenal infection, produces vast disruption in the body. As a result, the basic functions of the body are disabled. The body is even unable to maintain its natural balance. Water, for instance, can no longer be maintained at normal levels and is lost easily: the person exists in a permanent state of dehydration. Salt is also impossible to properly retain, and thus, sodium, as well as iodine, deficiency is common and persistent. This dehydration affects all tissues: there is a sort of dryness, even within the cells. The brain cells and spinal cord also become relatively dry. Thus, headaches, as well as stiff neck, are common. As this disruptive state continues, the first dire symptoms are a change in color of the skin and possibly mucous membranes. They become bronze. As the fluid levels drop further, weight loss may occur: blood pressure drops, the person becomes agitated, there may be nausea and vomiting, and the urine output declines. If uncontrolled, this may lead to potentially dire reactions, such as shock, or even death.

Prior to the development of treatment Addison's was routinely fatal. Then, it was discovered that an extract made from animal adrenal glands halted the crisis. Fishbein notes that hundreds of people who would otherwise have died were saved. Incredibly, the original treatments were natural extracts. These extracts have been systematically removed from the market by the drug powers. Yet, there are a number of other sources of equal power. This includes steroid concentrates, such as triple-strength royal jelly and raw maca root extract, which are highly used in the treatment of this condition.

Addison's usually develops over a prolonged period. When it strikes with its usual ferocity, it gives the appearance of an acute illness. However, this is merely the final stage of a prolonged illness. The fact is the majority of victims fail to realize they have this condition until it is too late. What's more, physicians are fully unaware of the early symptoms. Thus, they miss the diagnosis, usually deeming it as a psychological issue or stress. Or, they may diagnose some sort of disease, like GERD, migraine, hiatus hernia, esophagitis, spastic colon, yeast syndrome, chronic fatigue, fibromyalgia, depression, panic attacks, or similar vague illnesses, that disguise the cause. Yet, they never consider the real origin of these conditions, which is adrenal exhaustion.

Medical textbooks claim that Addison's or Addison's-like illnesses are rare. These textbooks are completely in error. In fact, tens of millions of Westerners, particularly Americans, suffer from at least a degree of Addison's disease and are ready victims for its more severe manifestations. This is particularly true if serious stressors occur or if faulty dietary habits are not halted.

Doctors simply are unaware of the physiology of this syndrome. Plus, another reason there is a failure to diagnose it is because for the mild to moderate forms doctors lack any cures. In contrast, there are numerous natural therapies which are effective. Doctors take a different approach. They have ready therapies for merely the symptoms of Addison's or, more correctly, sub-clinical or low level Addison's: heartburn, vague digestive complaints, depression, anxiety, nervousness, tiredness, and irritability. For these conditions drugs are usually prescribed. This is why innumerable cases are never diagnosed. The drugs conceal the symptoms, and no further investigations are performed. The drugs disguise the fact that these individuals suffer from adrenal collapse, not mere acid reflux, chronic fatigue, or mental disorders. All such symptoms are the result of the adrenal collapse. Thus, instead of merely a few bothersome symptoms which require symptomatic treatment, it is the adrenals or, rather, the entire endocrine system which much be treated.

Yet, regardless of the cause if the adrenals are weak or traumatized, they are highly vulnerable to infection. What's more, these weakened adrenals make the entire body vulnerable. In severe adrenal insufficiency infections can readily gain the advantage. In his medical encyclopedia Fishbein notes that in the untreated case "infections tend to become overwhelming. Complications can include progressive disability, weakness, and death." In fact, in such cases a relatively minor stress or infection can lead to dire consequences.

Again, it is critical to properly diagnose such an individual. There may be a mainly adrenal component with a degree of thyroid or pituitary element. Yet, with the primarily adrenal type caution must be exerted regarding the thyroid component. The intake of potent thyroid medicines can aggravate the condition, precipitating adrenal crisis. Thyroid hormone activates the nervous system. This may prove overpowering for the already depleted adrenals. Thus, efforts must be focused upon regenerating the adrenals, with additional effort to normalize the pituitary.

This vulnerability to infection of the adrenal type is a critical issue. This is because in order for such an individual to regain superb health the infections must be cleared. Currently, this is being achieved through the use of potent spice extracts. These are derived from wild or remote-grown spices, such as wild oregano and sage, as well as cumin and cinnamon. Spices have a vast history as germicides.

Recent research confirms that wild and remote-source spice extracts are the most potent naturally occurring germ killers known. By regularly taking spice extracts, such as wild oregano oil (Mediterranean source, hand-picked) and a combination of extracts of cumin, sage, bay leaf, and oregano, infections can be purged from the body. Here, a three-pronged therapy is ideal. This is the oil of wild oregano, the aromatic juice of wild oregano, and the aromatic four-spice compound as a desiccated wild spice extract capsule. In this regard the oregano juice is a particularly aggressive treatment. The crude herb, along with the anti-viral spice *Rhus coriaria*, may also be taken. The result is a dramatic improvement in health. For the severe adrenal case such a therapy may make the difference between life or death. Ideally, this multiple therapy is indicated, that is taking the oil under the tongue for direct absorption and for the head and neck, along with the juice and the multiple spice capsule orally. Then, for extra power the crude herb may be taken.

Multiple spice capsule therapy is based upon research at Georgetown Medical Center, where it was proven that the components of this capsule are capable of even killing drug-resistant germs. These extracts are in a base of extra virgin olive oil. They are also found in capsules as desiccated spice powders. This is the ideal way to administer the wild spice extracts in the treatment of chronic conditions.

The adrenal type can die from sudden stress reactions. Yet, this only occurs in the extreme. Even so, it is important to realize the vulnerability. This is the vulnerability to heat exhaustion, allergic shock, and sudden infection. The vulnerability to infection may be overlooked, simply because there has been a failure to determine the metabolic type. This could result in premature death. So, the critical issue is to determine if an adrenal disorder exists. This can be found through body conformation.

Key signs to look for also include crowding of the lower incisors, delicate frame (but not always), and thin or medium-thin hair. There may be a full head of hair, but the

144 The Body Shape Diet

strands are fine. The key one is the length of the fingers, the index versus the ring finger. With the adrenal type, usually, the index finger is longer than the ring finger or at least as long. Again, an obviously longer index finger is a clear evidence of adrenal syndrome. This occurs due to a lack of powerful steroids, known as androgens, which influence skeletal development. Further evidence of this type can be achieved through self-testing. The symptoms and signs of adrenal collapse are well published. Thus, all a person has to do is check the symptoms and add up the score. This is a reliable method for determining not only the existence of adrenal insufficiency but also its severity.

The following test will determine the degree of adrenal insufficiency. A hand-held or desk mirror may be helpful when taking this test.

Take the following test, adding one point per item, unless indicated otherwise. Which of these apply to you?

1. constant fatigue (2 points)
2. muscular weakness (2 points)
3. sweating or wetness of hands and feet
4. nervousness or sensations of apprehension
5. insomnia (2 points)
6. very low blood pressure (2 points)
7. thin appearance of the face
8. hair is thin (2 points)
9. chin is small, thin-boned, or receding (3 points)
10. dark or deep circles under the eyes
11. mood swings
12. paranoia
13. lightheaded sensation
14. cravings for salt (2 points)

15. cravings for sugar (2 points)
16. intolerance to fumes or cigarette smoke (2 points)
17. chronic stiffness of the neck or upper back (stiff spine)
18. hives and other rashes
19. vulnerable to food allergy reactions
20. generally weak (weak muscles)
21. get tired easily in the afternoon or after meals (2 points)
22. have no energy by the end of the day (2 points)
23. PMS
24. chronic heartburn
25. panic attacks (2 points)
26. hair is straight and fine (3 points)
27. unusually ticklish
28. hair loss on outer third of legs (2 points)
29. phobias
30. compulsive behavior
31. blood sugar disturbances
32. high sensitivity to noise (2 points)
33. easily frightened
34. easily frustrated
35. spastic neck
36. cold extremities
37. history of consuming large amounts of sugar (2 points)
38. feeling of being run down (2 points)
39. weak voice
40. weak heart or irregular pulse (palpitations)
41. easily distracted
42. tendency to have guilt feelings
43. clumsiness
44. skin has an unusual bronze color (2 points)
46. extremely sensitive to odors, perfume, and/or cigarette smoke

47. crowding of the lower incisors (3 points)
48. first finger is longer than the ring finger (4 points)
    —multiply times 2 if on both hands
49. first finger is equal in length to the ring finger (2 points)
    —multiply times two if on both hands
50. tendency to develop yeast or fungal infections
51. regularly use cortisone or prednisone (or used it heavily (2 points) in the past)
52. pigment spots on temple, upper back, palm, lips, or chest
53. easily develop lung or bronchial infections or TB (3 points)
54. eczema and/or psoriasis
55. blond hair and blue-eyed
56. poor concentration (2 points)
57. depression
58. fainting spells (2 points)
59. unusually sensitive to smells (2 points)
60. history of food allergies
61. second toe is longer than the big toe (2 points)
62. constantly feel urge to urinate but volume is low
63. cravings for chocolate
64. all senses very acute (2 points)
65. nervous habit of rolling or twisting things
66. vulnerable to viral infections, especially Epstein-Barr
67. loss of pigment on skin (vitiligo)

Your Score _____

Note: use the diagram, key signs, and the results of this test to make an assessment.

Anyone with a score above 6 has probable adrenal insufficiency, while a score from 7 to 14 indicates a mild-to-moderate case. A score from 15 to 21 indicates a moderate-to-severe case, while a score from 22 to 30 represents extreme adrenal exhaustion. A score from 31 to 37 is worrisome and represents profoundly extreme adrenal exhaustion, while a score above 38 is dire and represents potentially fatal adrenal collapse or at least the vulnerability for serious disease. Anyone who scores above 20 should be on a daily dose of high-grade royal jelly such as the 3x undiluted capsules fortified with rosemary and sage as well as the crude raw royal jelly paste emulsified in a base of cold-pressed pumpkinseed oil, the latter also providing valuable steroids. Also, a raw purple maca and blue corn extract should be consumed, about 20 drops twice daily, as well as wild- and remote-source vitamin C in the form of a purely-C complex (camu camu, acerola, and rose hips). Additionally, wild source salt capsules, with wild oregano, should be routinely consumed. So should wild saltgrass extract (see AmericanWildFoods.com).

The pituitary type (super-slow metabolizer)

A person who loves life, the pituitary type is perhaps the most challenging of all. This is because this type is an extreme example of endocrine dysfunction, perhaps the most extreme. In this type all the endocrine glands are dysfunctional. What's more, often, it takes a monumental effort to bring these glands into balance. Yet, surely, this can be achieved.

The pituitary type is rarely thin. Here, the metabolism is too slow, and so people with this type usually easily put on weight. In this type there is usually a prolonged history of weight problems, even beginning in childhood. The problem can also develop spontaneously, for instance, after trauma, pregnancy/childbirth, or surgery.

These people are often slow in everything they do. Yet, they are thorough. They may even be highly competent. It is just that, physically, they are slow or, rather, methodical. Even so, their minds may also be sluggish. So, both scenarios, an intelligent mind and a sluggish mind, are possible. In this type the shoulders are usually narrow or small. The head is also small compared to the rest of the body.

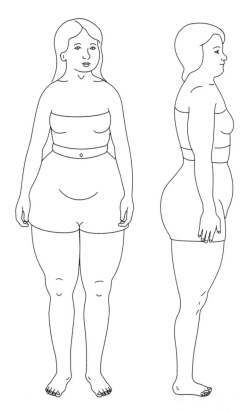

FIG. 6 Female pituitary body type

The most prominent portion of the body is often the buttocks, which can be enormous. The hips are also usually large. Yet, the waist (above the hips) can be small. The abdomen, too, is prominent. In fact, this may be the most prominent feature.

These people rarely have a true beer belly. It is more of an obesity problem, with the fat being concentrated on the lower abdomen, buttocks, hips, and thighs. There may even be accumulations of fat on the arms, about the shoulders, around the wrists and elbows, and around the knees. This

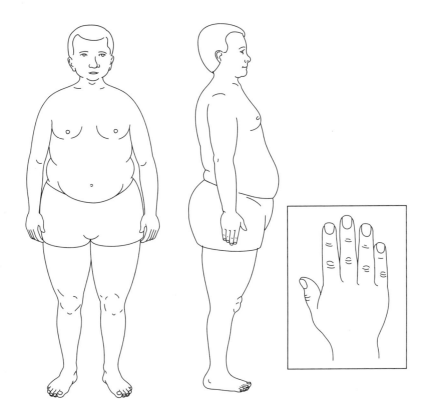

FIG. 7 Male pituitary body type

person rarely 'becomes' obese. It is a hormonal weakness, which causes this. It is an inherited problem. In some cases there can be a kind of round center to the abdomen, like a huge bloated circle.

This person is not naturally huge. In other words, the frame of such a person is often delicate. Usually, he or she has a fine bone structure, which means this body is not made to be heavy. Yet, this would almost never be realized due to this amount of swelling and fat deposition. In men the fat may concentrate in the abdomen. Yet, again, the buttocks may be relatively fat. In women the fat is heavily concentrated about the hips and thighs as well as the buttocks. Incredibly, usually, despite this significant weight the hands and feet are small, even tiny. Any person with a round head plus unusually tiny feet or hands likely has a pituitary disorder.

There is another pituitary type. Here, the head may actually be normal or even large. This type may be due to overactivity of the glands, a syndrome of excessive pituitary activity. In this sub-type the hands and feet are obviously large. In particular, the fingers are long, although the palm may also be long. This is the most rare of the two types.

Those pituitary types with long hands, large feet, and big bones should follow essentially the thyroid type diet. They can modify this slightly by also eating seafood and taking essential fatty acid supplements. For this type both undiluted royal jelly capsules and the thyroid-supporting northern Pacific kelp plus rosemary and wild oregano capsules should be consumed. So should wild raw eight berries drops and the hydrosols of wild rosemary and oregano. Also, the vitamin A/D-rich wild sockeye salmon oil should also be consumed.

For the sluggish pituitary type the neck region is characteristic. At its back there is a fat pad around the lower part. The nose is also usually short, in other words, it is rarely long and thin. Pituitary types often have a pug nose. The tip is usually rounded. The nose may also be slightly uplifted. The face gives a sort of 'baby face' appearance, which is why such people might be regarded as happy-go-lucky. The neck itself is usually short. The lips, while short, are usually full. As described by Benedict the typical look and expressions of this type are child-like, which is why pituitary types usually look much younger than their age. This is true only of those with underactive pituitaries. Again, regarding the neck in some individuals it is so short that it is as if there is no neck, somewhat like the appearance, for instance, of Winston Churchill.

The hands are characteristic. In addition to their small size compared to the size of the person they are plump. Instead of prominent bony knuckles there are dimples. Again, pituitary types have tiny heads and big bodies

The brain controls all functions. One of the most significant components of this organ is the pituitary. This is such an important system that it is given its own special protective bony tissue, known as the sella tursica. Yet, it is a relatively small endocrine gland, being about the size of a large pea. Regardless, it has a massive influence on the body. This gland is located in the front of the brain, in fact, behind the eyes at the base of the brain. It consists of two parts, the anterior and posterior lobes. The posterior part is largely a derivative of nerve tissue from the brain, while the anterior part is a derivative of blood vessel tissue.

People with the brain-pituitary syndrome suffer a significant dilemma: their brain chemistry is usually sluggish.

Their entire nervous systems are out of balance, which negatively affects all organ function. In fact, in many cases none of these organ systems seem to work. The metabolic rate is exceedingly slow. Doctors don't know what to do with them, often abandoning them in complete frustration. Yet, it is far from an impossible problem, if the proper approach is taken. Even so, without vigorous treatment it is often difficult to gain normalization of function. This can only be achieved by massive intervention in the form of strict dietary changes plus the intake of high-grade plant oils and nutritional supplements.

The intake of plant oils is critical. The ideal plant oils include pure, organic Amazonian sacha inchi oil. This is harvested in a way that supports the growth of the Amazon. This is exclusively available in the blue and yellow label brand. Cold-pressed, remote-grown sesame oil, cold-pressed black seed oil, and cold-pressed pumpkinseed oil are also invaluable.

The ideal type of sacha inchi oil must be organically grown and cold-pressed. This is from the seed pods, which are organically grown in the Amazon near the Peruvian border. The intake of this oil highly boosts pituitary function. This is because it is a rich source of a wide range of nutrients. Additionally, people with pituitary syndrome often suffer from skin disorders. Here, cold-pressed sacha inchi oil is invaluable. It is well known that the natives of the Amazon, who consume this oil and seed, have magnificent skin. This is because sacha inchi oil, rich in vitamin E, beta carotene, and amino acids, is highly nourishing to both the skin and the glands. Regardless, the skin itself is an endocrine gland.

Fish is a healthy pituitary food. It also contains the ideal types of amino acids for pituitary function. Yet, there is a warning. In particular, for pituitary types the intake of ocean fish due to mercury contamination must be curbed. Mercury greatly poisons this gland. Also, sacha inchi oil, being pure and unrefined, is preferable as a source of omega-3s versus highly refined and adulterated fish oils. Note: there are types of fatty fish available which are low in mercury. These higher quality fish can be consumed more vigorously than the commercial types. (See www.AmericanWildFoods.com.)

Commercial fish oils should be avoided. This is because they are too refined. In particular, people with pituitary types should avoid the intake of the so-called pharmaceutical-grade fish oils. These highly refined oils contain residues of detergents. Essentially, they are no longer natural and, rather, are a type of chemical supplement. In contrast, the truly organically grown sacha inchi oil is crude cold-pressed, completely natural and free of chemicals. It is essentially a vegetable fish oil replacement. In this regard it provides the precursors for the creation of fish oils.

There is another option which must be considered. This is wild sockeye salmon oil. This is derived from remote-source northern Alaskan fish. The oil is made from a kind of crude process, merely steam-distilled. There is no other processing involved. No detergents or chemicals are used. Tests prove that, because of the remote-source and the relatively small size of the fish, the oil is extremely low in heavy metals and/or contaminants. This is why no further refinement is required. Thus, it is the ideal whole fish oil source for pituitary types. In fact, it is ideal for all people. This is available as a crude oil (unfiltered and unrefined) in eight ounce bottles or 500 milligram fish gelatin capsules. A bonus is that in contrast to commercial fish oil capsules wild Alaskan sockeye salmon is an excellent source of vitamins

A and D. Both these vitamins are direly needed for normal functioning of the endocrine glands, particularly the pituitary, thyroid, and adrenals. In contrast, for pituitary types, refined fish oil or so-called pharmaceutical grade fish oils are not advisable. These contain residues of chemicals used in refinement, which may poison the pituitary.

Also, food concentrates rich in chromium are ideal for this type. Examples include Peruvian purple corn drops and red sour grape powder. Rice bran also contains a significant amount of chromium. Regarding the latter this will aid greatly in firming up the body and helping to strengthen the muscles. Red sour grape also contains hormone-like substances from grape skins, which help strengthen the pituitary. This includes the hormone/polyphenol known as resveratrol, which is highly potent for the balancing of the pituitary gland. In particular, for pituitary types, who suffer from high blood pressure, the latter two supplements are indispensable. The same is true of those types, where there is dense fat deposition along the sides of the body and buttocks. Crude chromium and resveratrol, as found in red sour grape powder, help mobilize these fat stores.

Pituitary types are in love with life. They are often jovial and, usually, fun to be around. They tend to be self-deprecating. This is largely because of low self image due to their appearance. Even so, they love to have fun. They love positive stimuli. They are rarely hurtful to others. However, they may belittle themselves. Sweet people are rarely violent. Rather, usually, they may themselves be victims of violence. Yet, despite their inherent happiness and easy-going nature, their ill health interferes with true pleasure. One pleasure they often pursue is eating, which they may do with recklessness. Usually, they eat the wrong foods, notably greasy foods, refined starches, oily (refined) salty snacks, and sweets. They can handle a great deal of food and only rarely complain of digestive disorders. Often, this is their "only enjoyment," while, sadly, they fail to realize that such foods perpetuate their misery.

There are specific signs and symptoms of sluggish pituitary function. To determine a person's specific status a test can be performed. Such a written test has never before been available. Now, the individual can determine if his/her problem is primarily or partially pituitary, that is without invasive or dangerous tests.

Take the following test to determine your degree of pituitary dysfunction:

1. chronically overweight
2. smaller than normal uterus, ovaries, or testes (3 points)
3. unusually small penis (3 points)
4. fat pads around the ankle bones (2 points)
5. highly sensitive to perfumes/chemicals (2 points)
6. extreme fat deposits around the buttocks (2 points)
7. fat deposits about or below the neck, hump-like (3 points)
8. impotence, infertility, or lack of sexual desire (2 points)
9. unable to generate sex desire (2 points)
10. child-like or weak voice (2 points)
11. persistent headaches
12. easily exhausted
13. skin which is white and blotched (alabaster-like)
14. low body temperature
15. sluggish metabolism (2 points)
16. sluggish digestion
17. irregular menstruation or scant menstruation (2 points)

18. complete lack of menstruation (3 points)
19. extremities are constantly cold
20. lack of hair growth on body or scalp (2 points)
21. unusually prominent forehead
22. pendulous abdomen (2 points)
23. pear-shaped figure (3 points)
24. hands are long, with tapering fingers
25. delicate, fine skin
26. for males: feminine body type (2 points)
27. round, chubby face (2 points)
28. lips project outward (2 points)
29. small or pug nose (3 points)
30. fine, clear facial skin
31. fine hair
32. scant eyelashes (2 points)
33. large round cheeks, which are prominent
34. under-developed skeleton (small bone frame for size)
35. short and chubby neck (2 points)
36. droopy skin on inside of thighs
37. round or fatty limbs (2 points)
38. layer of fat over the entire body (2 points)
39. lack of hair everywhere except head (3 points)
40. mind works slowly
41. heavy amount of fat in the buttocks, where they appear dimpled (that is in women) - 2 points
42. weigh 300 to 400 pounds on a small or medium frame (3 points)
43. weigh over 400 pounds on a small or medium frame (5 points)
44. vitiligo that is loss of pigment from the skin (2 points)
45. skin and muscle droops from back of arm (also cellulite in this region—2 points)

46. cellulite along the outer thighs (2 points)
47. unusually small hands and feet (2 points)
48. pain behind the eye or in forehead
49. unusually small nail region on the fifth finger (2 points)

Your score _____

Note: use the diagram, key signs, and the results of this test to make an assessment.

A score of 3 to 8 indicates mild-to-moderate pituitary syndrome, while a score from 9 to 16 indicates a moderate-to-severe case. A score of 17 to 25 demonstrates a severe or rather extreme case, while a score from 26 to 32 indicates a profoundly extreme case. Any score above 34 is a sign of dire pituitary disorder and may be a warning of pituitary tumor. Such a score is an example of extreme collapse of the endocrine system.

The pituitary type may be easily confused with the thyroid and adrenal types. Never make a quick decision regarding the type. Thus, individuals must study the various types until they determine which one fits best. It may not always be a perfect fit. Determine it as close as possible. There are at least three variations of this type, most of which have already been listed.

Usually, people with pituitary imbalance are incorrectly diagnosed as being hypothyroid. While hypothyroidism is a definite factor, it isn't the primary one. In such individuals it is the pituitary which is truly dysfunctional, with thyroid, ovarian, adrenal, and/or testicular imbalances being secondary. In this condition the entire endocrine system is imbalanced. Effort must be made to return balance to this system, so that the individual can live a relatively normal life. This usually requires aggressively changing the diet, increasing the intake of high-grade, unprocessed fatty acids, and taking the appropriate nutritional supplements.

The diet in this instance must be moderate in meat products, emphasizing wild game, fish, and poultry. Seafood is also acceptable. The meat must be organic, and the fish and seafood must be wild. Natural, wild whitefish is an ideal food for this type. However, it may be necessary to avoid bottom feeding fish, such as flounder and sole, which may be too high in toxins that can disrupt the function of the gland. Other fish to avoid, which are exceedingly high in toxins, include swordfish, marlin, albacore tuna, bluefish, and King Salmon.

Wild animals (or farm-raised wild-like animals) are the ideal meat for these individuals. Any animal which uses its muscles extensively, like ducks, quail, pheasant, bison, deer, and elk, must rely on various muscle-empowering hormones. These hormones are concentrated in the meat and when this flesh is eaten, the benefits are procured.

Milk products may be well tolerated. The occasional intake of goat's and sheep's yogurt is acceptable. Nuts and seeds are ideal foods, especially hormone-rich pine nuts, almonds, filberts, and walnuts. Vegetables and fruit can be eaten relatively freely, but high-sugar fruit must be strictly avoided. Thus, apples, pears, grapes, pineapple, and dried fruit should be eliminated from the diet. The preferred fruit are melons, grapefruit, lemons, limes, papaya, and strawberries as well as blueberries, cranberries, blackberries, and black raspberries.

Pomegranate may prove invaluable, as this improves blood flow to the brain. This can be consumed as a pure juice or preferably as a sour concentrate. Another powerful extract for the pituitary is organic black mulberry juice, which greatly boosts this organ's chemistry (again, available as a special internet purchase). Wild blueberry juice is also ideal, available under the brands Van Dykes and Wyman's, which may be found on the internet or in select health food stores. Yet, in some instances, where there is extreme fungal overload, all fruit may need to be eliminated, at least temporarily.

Starchy foods must be strictly avoided. No bread of any kind is allowed. Deep fried foods must also be strictly avoided, as these greatly interfere with hormone metabolism. Nuts and seeds are ideal, since they contain small amounts of natural hormones and are a rich source of certain vitamins and minerals. However, the key in this condition is to eat plenty of meat as well as fish. Regarding fish the fatty ones are ideal, for instance, salmon and halibut. Sardines and herring are also ideal foods. Only wild fish are allowed. One exception is truly organic farm raised fish fed wild-like feed. The best seafood is lobster and crab. People with this type should ideally eat a helping or two of these seafood every week. These shellfish are top sources of naturally occurring hormones. If eating any such fish regularly, be sure to take a purging agent, such as those mentioned in this book, to decontaminate mercury residues.

Even so, many pituitary types are allergic to seafood, so it must be eaten to tolerance. Also, again, there is the issue of contamination of the ocean with toxic chemicals and heavy metals. So, eat such food reasonably.

Eggs are allowed. Only organic or free-range eggs must be used. Look in specialty stores for quail eggs. These are particularly rich in hormones. This is the ideal type of eggs to consume. When cooking eggs, ideally, keep the yolks soft, since this keeps the naturally occurring hormones intact. The best fruit are olives and avocados, as they contain a variety of fat soluble hormone-like substances.

Pituitary types should never eat wheat. Rye should also be avoided. These gluten-rich grains are too difficult to digest for individuals with such slow metabolism. Optionally, wild rice and potatoes with the skin on are acceptable. Brown rice can be eaten in moderation but should be combined with wild rice. Other healthy carbohydrate sources might include amaranth, teff, and quinoa. Often, such individuals crave bread, rolls, and wheat-based foods. They may eat as much as a loaf of bread per day. Plus, they often binge on crackers, eating an entire box in a sitting. Dinner rolls are another weakness. The fact is the breadbasket is their doom.

Such foods are highly addictive, not just for taste but also chemically. For instance, wheat contains a substance which mimics insulin. In fact, this substance binds to brain cell receptors, causing a temporary mood elevation. However, soon thereafter this results in a lowering of blood sugar levels, which may cause both depression and fatigue. What's more, the majority of commercial wheat products contain partially hydrogenated and/or hydrogenated oils, which greatly interfere with pituitary function.

The action of wheat on the brain can be profound. This is because it contains a number of substances with morphine-like activity. Pituitary types often have mood imbalances, so they will crave or eat anything which acts as a stimulant.

Thus, allergenic foods are craved, because they cause a temporary boost in endorphin levels. The 'wheat high,' however, is only temporary. Wheat-based foods are repeatedly consumed to regain it. This explains the addiction. After the high there is usually a crash, leading, ultimately, to further binging. In this situation it is not possible to have 'a little bit.' Any amount is too much, since this may rapidly revive the addiction.

For pituitary types all wheat products or wheat-containing foods must be strictly eliminated. For ideal results rye, barley, and oats should also be eliminated. Even so, in some instances, oat bran cereal may be well tolerated. It is low in carbohydrates and relatively low in brain-stimulating agents. Rice bran is also acceptable. As sources of starch brown rice and wild rice are superior to grains, since these foods are less toxic and more readily digested. Other sources of starch which are usually well tolerated include baked organic potatoes, organic sweet potatoes, organic squash, amaranth, and quinoa. Ideally, the sweet potatoes and potatoes should be eaten raw or cooked moderately.

For this type refined sugar is devastating. All foods containing it must be avoided. Sugar is highly destructive to the hormones, and pituitary types must conserve all their hormone reserve, which is limited. Sugar depletes this reserve. It destroys hormones by oxidizing them. Plus, it directly poisons the glands, especially the adrenals and pituitary. When the intake of sugar is high, hormone synthesis greatly decreases. Hormones are made from amino acids, that is protein residues, as well as fatty acids: never sugar. These proteins and fatty acids are derived from truly nutritious food, the kind of food which is rarely eaten by sugar addicts. Thus, by replacing healthier caloric sources sugar impedes hormone production. It also directly destroys key vitamins needed for pituitary and adrenal function. These vitamins, which are readily destroyed by sugar, include thiamine, niacin, pantothenic acid, folic acid, and vitamin C.

Vaccines are another destructive factor. In fact, multiple vaccinations can actually cause this syndrome. This is partly due to the toxic substances found in these vaccines. It is also due to the poisonous germs transmitted by these injections. Particularly in the early era of vaccination, 1950 through 2003, vaccines were heavily laden with mercury. Since then public scrutiny caused the pharmaceutical houses to decrease the amount of mercury used in these injections. Another source of contamination is mercury in dental fillings. This places the mercury in the most dire place possible, which is directly near the brain and, therefore, the pituitary. Vaccines are the most common cause of pituitary disruption, followed by mercury amalgam fillings. Insecticide and pesticide intoxication may also corrupt this gland.

Mercury is an extreme pituitary poison. So is formaldehyde, a virtually universal vaccine additive. Then, these substances were/are injected directly into the bloodstream of the victims, and as a result the toxins were/are concentrated in the brain, particularly the pituitary gland. Even more dire are the microbes, in particular, vaccine viruses. These viruses are neurologically active, that is they readily enter the brain and other neurological tissues. The pituitary is a part of the nervous system. Incredibly, mercury readily passes through this barrier. Furthermore, this poisonous metal weakens the blood-brain barrier, making the tissues more vulnerable to viral invasion. Thus, a vast number of individuals with the pituitary type are victims of vaccination.

As vaccines weaken immunity the body is left vulnerable to invasion by opportunists. One of these opportunists is the fungi. This group of germs includes yeasts. As mentioned previously people with chronic endocrine disorders are vulnerable to chronic infection. In fact, yeast infections are a common dilemma in people with sluggish pituitary function, particularly those who have received multiple vaccinations. Actually, people with the pituitary type who constantly crave sugar are likely infested with yeast. The fungus can actually attack the pituitary gland itself. Thus, it must be systematically purged from the body. Exposure to mercury accelerates the growth of such fungi. Radiation therapy also increases fungal growth. Another factor is stress, which can not only weaken the function of the endocrine glands, particularly the pituitary, but also increase the risks for fungal and viral syndromes.

Pituitary types are in dire need of hormones. They cannot afford any depletion of their reserves, not even a molecule. This is because of all metabolic types the pituitary type is the most direly deficient in hormones. Plus, people with this type have a difficult time generating new hormones. Their metabolism is simply too slow. So, they must conserve any hormones and avoid all crises. They do so by methodically planning all they do. This is a protective reflex and is absolutely normal. Yet, unfortunately many such individuals have been regarded abnormal by the medical profession and treated with medication; some have been institutionalized. Yet, these poor souls were only doing what their bodies demanded of them, which is protecting themselves from their weaknesses.

Pituitary damage is largely the consequence of the high sugar diet. A careful history will reveal that people with pituitary disorders often have a history of being major sweet and sugar consumers, either when younger and even currently. Plus, their parents were usually sugar addicts. Or, one or both of the parents may have been an alcoholic. The highly toxic effects of alcohol on brain tissue are well known. Yet, what is little know is that the pituitary, which is largely brain tissue, is direly damaged by alcohol. In fact, this toxin shrinks this gland. This toxicity is particularly dire for the developing fetus. For the fetus any amount of alcohol will poison, even destroy, this gland. Thus, Fetal Alcohol Syndrome is largely a consequence of the destruction of the pituitary. Pituitary types should touch not a drop of alcohol. They should even avoid alcohol-based drugs and herbs.

In a pregnant mother as little as a drink a day or every other day is sufficient to damage the infant's pituitary. Heavy drinkers, that is those who drink two or more alcoholic beverages per day, greatly place the fetus at risk, not only for weak pituitary syndrome but also for serious and permanent brain damage. Even males who drink place their offspring at risk. Sperm is readily damaged by alcohol. If a damaged sperm unites with an ovum, the resulting baby can suffer significant brain damage, including damage to the pituitary. A list of substances and/or foods which destroy or deplete pituitary hormones includes:

- refined sugar
- corn syrup
- food dyes
- artificial flavors
- artificial sweeteners, particularly NutraSweet
- white flour

- white rice
- acetaminophen
- cholesterol-lowering agents (that is statins)
- mineral oil
- caffeine
- MSG
- sulfites
- formaldehyde
- lead
- mycotoxins (mold toxins)
- vaccines
- cortisone (prednisone)
- drugs
- theobromine (as found in cocoa and chocolate)

Substances/nutrients which help preserve hormones include natural vitamin C (as found in natural extracts of camu camu, acerola, and rose hips), natural vitamin E (sunflower seed source), natural-source beta carotene, flavonoids, organic acids, wild oregano oil, wild rosemary oil, chelated zinc, vitamin B_6, riboflavin, and pantothenic acid. Of these, natural-source vitamin E is a key substance for preserving hormones, especially those arising from the pituitary. Sunflower seed vitamin E complex is ideal, since it is well tolerated and readily absorbed. Be sure to procure the type emulsified in crude pumpkinseed oil and wild red palm oil. Regardless, vitamin E helps prevent the oxidation of pituitary hormones.

Another key substance is wild rosemary oil. This oil has a predilection for brain tissue. It is the ideal substance for conserving the hormones of the brain, that is the hormones of the pituitary, pineal, and hypothalamus. There is also good evidence that rosemary oil preserves the adrenal glands. Interestingly, in aromatherapy rosemary oil has long been regarded as an agent for balancing, as well as strengthening, the adrenal glands. The ideal form for this substance is as an emulsion (sublingual drops) in extra virgin olive oil derived from the wild Mediterranean species. For hormone health both sunflower seed oil vitamin E and wild rosemary oil should ideally be taken as sublingual drops.

Only natural substances preserve hormones. Natural vitamin E and beta carotene are powerful preservatives. These vitamins are found in rich amounts in crude red palm oil, cold-pressed Austrian pumpkinseed oil. Regarding vitamin E, cold-pressed Austrian pumpkinseed oil and mountain-grown sesame oil are also rich. Crude sour grape extracts, as well as muscadine grape skin powder, are potent sources of hormones. This is particularly true of the powders, which are concentrates of the hormone-rich skins. A high-grade muscadine powder, as found on the internet (Americanwildfoods.com) or in stores, is another means to naturally boost the hormone glands, particularly the pituitary. Another powerful source of hormone-like substances are the skins of wild berries. Concentrates of these skins are also available in a potent form, that is as raw wild berry drops.

Hormones are made primarily from amino acids, although a few are made from lipids. Regarding the latter it is mainly the adrenal and sex hormones which are lipids. Cholesterol is the major lipid used in the synthesis of these hormones. Animal foods are the only dietary source of cholesterol. In fact, animals are synthetic factories for this substance. This is why such foods must form the primary source of calories in this diet. Thus, healthy sources of cholesterol—animal foods—must be included in the diet. These include organic whole milk, especially raw/unpastuerized, as well as yogurt, kefir, quark, and eggs. All such foods must be consumed from pure unadulterated sources.

Admittedly, some individuals are allergic to milk products. Usually, this is a cow's milk allergy. I have found that the allergy can often be neutralized through the intake of oil of wild oregano (in extra virgin olive oil, blue label hand-picked and wild). Also, this allergic tendency is reduced when consuming raw organic milk. In most instances a few drops of the oil of wild oregano or oil of edible clove buds added to the milk neutralizes any allergy. Wild oregano crude herbal capsules with Rhus coriaria are also anti-allergy. To neutralize the allergic potential a few capsules may be taken with each meal. Also, goat's and sheep's milk products are excellent options.

Even so, for the pituitary type milk products are of modest value. In some of these people severe intolerance to milk, that is cow's milk, is evident. Thus, in most instances milk products are restricted, perhaps, except goat's and sheep's milk products. Feta cheese may be tolerated, since it is highly digestible. In some pituitary types this may be consumed freely, as it is a valuable source of natural hormones, fat soluble vitamins, minerals, and amino acids.

Like all organs the pituitary is in dire need of certain nutrients. Amino acids feed it, since the majority of pituitary hormones are derived from them. Thus, normal function of this gland is dependent upon an adequate supply of nutrients. In particular, certain vitamins and minerals play a key role. The primary vitamins required by this organ include vitamin A, vitamin C, riboflavin, that is vitamin B_2, vitamin B_6, folic acid, and vitamin E. The main minerals are zinc, selenium, and magnesium. Yet, of all nutrients the absolutely key ones are vitamin A, riboflavin, vitamin C, B_6, niacin, essential fatty acids, vitamin E (ideally from sunflower seed oil), and zinc. Try to get the nutrients from truly natural sources. Synthetic nutrients are not as effective as are the natural ones and are, in fact, toxic.

The essential fatty acids are crucial for pituitary gland health. The ideal ones are derived from wild seeds or various fruit/nut seeds. One of the finest sources is the cold-pressed oil of sacha inchi seed. This seed is organically grown in the Amazon. This is a medicinal type of fatty seed, which is some 52% omega-3s by weight. This means sacha inchi oil is the most dense source of omega-3s known. The types of omega-3s found in sacha inchi oil are the ideal types for conversion into the all-important long chain fatty acids, EPA and DHA.

Whenever taking large amounts of essential fatty acids and various nut/seed oils, it is crucial to increase the intake of natural-source vitamin E. Be aware that all soy-based vitamin E supplements are derived from genetically engineered soy beans. The latter contain poisonous compounds. These fake soybeans are engineered to produce pesticides. These pesticides are found in the end product. Thus, commercial soy products, including soybean oil-derived vitamin E, are poisonous. Vitamin E from sunflower seed oil is a healthy option.

The pituitary gland consumes a significant amount of the body's supplies of the aforementioned nutrients. In fact, a severe deficiency of essential fatty acids leads to potentially permanent damage of this gland, greatly upsetting the chemistry of the entire body. In most instances pituitary types suffer from severe essential fatty acid deficiency. This accounts for the emphasis in this book on the intake of essential fatty acids-rich food as well as supplements. Again, the top food source of these fatty acids includes wild game, fatty fish, nuts, seeds, nut/seed oils (unrefined), crude pumpkinseed oil, flaxseed, berry seed essential fatty acids, sacha inchi seeds/oil, and purslane. Unless a person regularly eats such foods or takes such food supplements deficiency is inevitable.

Carbohydrates, especially the refined type, are the pituitary's doom. People with this type lack any capacity to burn such fuel. There is only one destination: fat cells. When carbohydrates are digested, they are converted to sugar in the form of glucose. In the normal individual the glucose is burned into fuel, or it is stored in the liver as glycogen. In the pituitary type the glucose is rarely burned, so there is only one other destination: the fat cells. However, with special therapy the ability of such a person to burn glucose may be enhanced. This is most effective when combined with eliminating the consumption of refined carbohydrates. If the person continues to eat sugar and starch, inevitably, much weight is gained. Also, the chemistry of the pituitary is disturbed. Yet, the multiple spice extract, combined with the grape skin concentrates, is so effective that a reasonable intake of whole carbohydrates is well tolerated. Also, wild berries and wild berry drops are starch blockers.

Again, the slow metabolism demands a reduction in carbohydrate intake. For carbohydrates the intake of fruits and vegetables is sufficient. Wild rice and alternative 'grains,' teff, quinoa, and amaranth, are usually well tolerated and offer much needed variety. Plus, again, a multiple spice complex made of researched-tested spice oils will naturally balance carbohydrate metabolism. In fact, incredibly a good carbohydrate meal may be consumed with impunity when taking such supplements.

Carbohydrate intolerance is known as syndrome X. It is a true endocrine or metabolic syndrome. Here, excess insulin drives glucose, a breakdown product of dietary starches and sugars, into the liver and fat cells, where it is synthesized into fat globules. This fat ultimately permeates all tissues, leading to various diseases, particularly cardiovascular disorders. This is the inevitable result of those addictive starches so loved by the pituitary type (the syndrome is also common in the thyroid types). Yet, virtually all doctors miss the issue with this syndrome. This is because they never determine the endocrine type, which is the key to preventing and reversing this syndrome.

The pituitary type thrives best when the insulin mechanism is normalized. This can largely be achieved through diet. However, the intake of a multiple spice extract for regulating blood sugar is crucial. Such a potent compound is ideal for the pituitary type. This is because it eliminates insulin resistance. In fact, these spice extracts balance the blood sugar rapidly by acting as a sort of natural insulin. Such substances boost pancreatic function, making insulin work better and even bolstering insulin production. This results in a vast improvement of the health of the pancreas.

Chromium is also readily absorbed in a natural and biological form. The ideal form is within food complexes. This is because chromium in isolation—the so-called inorganic type—is nearly impossible to absorb. It would be like trying to digest the chromium (chrome) used to make car bumpers. It, therefore, must be in a bound form to absorb. Two such complexes are the chromium chelates found in red sour grape and purple corn. Here, the chromium is bound to various organic substances and, thus, is readily absorbed. In contrast, a typical mineral supplement is poorly absorbed if at all.

Chromium boosts insulin synthesis. It also eradicates fatty liver. This is through causing the aggressive cellular burning of fat. Crude red sour grape contains a particularly rich amount of this nutrient. A mere two teaspoons provides over two-thirds the minimum daily requirement of this mineral. Purple corn is also rich in this mineral and contains it in a liquid form, as drops under the tongue. Such natural chromium is a vitality factor, helping to bolster the health of the pancreas as well as adrenals and pituitary.

Natural-source chromium is critical for the pituitary. This substance has a potent protective action on this gland, greatly reducing its stress. Also, sour grape flavonoids dramatically improve blood flow to the brain. Additionally, these flavonoids act as natural pituitary-like hormones.

The function of the pituitary is dependent upon a steady supply of energy. This is through blood glucose. The regular intake of natural chromium helps maintain proper blood sugar control. So do B vitamins. An excellent source of these B vitamins is the rice bran/polish mix, combined with torula yeast and royal jelly. This is available as a purely B complex powder free of all additives. This truly natural B complex supplement is found in superior health food stores. Also, pure organic rice bran, a tasty product, can be purchased either at health food stores or on the internet.

Natural-source B vitamins are direly needed by the pituitary. These include thiamine, niacin, riboflavin, choline, pyridoxine, folic acid, and B_{12}. Here, synthetic B vitamins found in the typical B complex supplement or multiple vitamin are of little or no value. Rather, it is the natural divinely-made vitamins that are truly effective. Again, such biologically active vitamins are found naturally, particularly in organic meat, whole grains, wild rice, royal jelly, food yeasts, and in concentrated form in the polish and bran of brown rice.

Crude rice polish and bran concentrates, combined with torula yeast and royal jelly powder, can be taken supplementally. This is the top source also of naturally occurring thiamine, niacin, choline, and biotin. The addition of royal jelly boosts the content of pantothenic acid, riboflavin, and pyridoxine.

There are many who claim that their vitamin pills are truly natural. They may even claim these pills, including multiple vitamins, are from food. This is impossible. There is no way to concentrate that amount of natural vitamins or minerals in such pills. This is a marketing tactic. Here, the actual sources are described. These are true sources. Additionally, the amounts are in modest doses. Yet, the biological activity is exceedingly high. Additionally, as is obvious a number of supplements must be taken to procure natural-source vitamins and minerals. There is no 'one-pill' answer.

B_{12} and folic acid are supplied mainly in red meat, poultry, egg yolk, cheese, yogurt, and fatty fish. Thus, a formula for procuring sufficient quantities of natural B complex is:

- crude rice polish/bran plus red sour grape and flaxseed
  - 3 to 4 heaping tablespoons daily

- royal jelly paste made from undiluted raw royal jelly and crude pumpkinseed oil - 1/2 teaspoon daily
- undiluted 3x royal jelly capsules - 2 to 4 daily
- wild greens concentrate - 1 teaspoon daily
- organic whole egg yolks - one or two daily
- crude red sour grape - one heaping teaspoonful daily
- purple corn drops (remote-source) - 50 or more drops daily

There is also the purely natural B complex supplement made from torula yeast, rice bran, and powdered royal jelly. This supplies the majority of the needed proportions. Additionally, it is a good idea to occasionally consume a raw organic egg. Don't worry about the milligram doses. These sources provide significant but modest doses. Yet, rather than the quantity it is the quality, in fact, the biological activity that matters.

Foods rich in chromium include the skins of red grapes, brewers yeast, blackstrap molasses, and egg yolks. This is why the regular intake of crude red sour grape powder, as well as muscadine powder and purple corn drops, is so crucial. An ideal way to get a daily natural dose of chromium is to eat two to three eggs over easy sprinkled heavily with a teaspoon or more of red sour grape powder. Top sources of B complex include the germ of whole grains, rice polish/bran, organic red meats, dark green leafy vegetables, egg yolks, yogurt, almonds, liver, and fatty fish.

With pituitary syndromes infection is a significant issue. This gland can be infected by a wide range of germs–bacteria, viruses, yeasts, molds and parasites. Such infections are usually chronic, and thus, predictably, they are rarely diagnosed. Toxicity is another factor. Brain tissue is highly vulnerable to the noxious effects of synthetic chemicals, and the pituitary is particularly sensitive. Heavy alcohol consumption especially damages it. Alcohol directly disrupts this gland. Food additives, especially aspartame, food dyes, sulfites, and MSG, readily poison it. The daily intake of aspartame, that is NutraSweet, is a primary cause of pituitary insufficiency. Obviously, prescription drugs and, particularly, street drugs are a major cause of pituitary damage. Signs and symptoms of pituitary toxicity include extreme sensitivity to cold, lowered body temperature, sluggish metabolism, poor reflexes, intolerance to exercise, cold extremities, weight disturbances, excruciating headaches, pain behind the eye, and exhaustion. These symptoms may also indicate poisoning by toxic compounds, particularly solvents, heavy metals, insecticides, herbicides, and drugs. To revive the function of this gland these substances must be purged from the body. This is through the use of a wild-source purging agent consisting of wild raw greens, black seed oil, extra virgin olive oil, raw cider vinegar, and spice oils. Wild raw dandelion greens and burdock greens or their extracts are particularly potent as a purge.

Thyroid-adrenal type

There are two main combination types. These are the thyroid-adrenal and adrenal-thyroid types. Other less common combination types include the thyroid-muscular (that is muscular-pancreatic), and pituitary-thyroid-adrenal. Of all these types the thyroid-adrenal is the most common. Thus, it is listed as one of the four main types. Next in frequency is the adrenal-thyroid type.

In modern medicine virtually all methods are rigid. A person has a thyroid or an adrenal problem separately, never in combination. This is the great fault of the medical system, to neglect completely the natural interactions of the body.

In medicine illnesses or syndromes are put into isolated categories. Yet, as has been made abundantly clear regarding the hormone system, the endocrine glands work as a team. Thus, it would be expected that people will have multiple dysfunctions. Even so, the important issue is to determine the primary types and the main dysfunctions. While in medicine combined disorders are neglected there is a definite syndrome combining both these types. In fact, in many cases whenever there is a thyroid disorder there is also an accompanying adrenal or pituitary component. The same is also true in reverse, that is individuals with primary adrenal problems often have a corresponding minor to moderate thyroid imbalance. Even so, virtually always one of these organ systems predominates.

Usually, in the thyroid-adrenal type there is a slight domination of the thyroid over the adrenal. Thus, emphasis should be placed upon treating the thyroid, the adrenal treatment being supportive. Yet, for ideal results both systems must be treated. Thus, it is important to realize that everyone has at least a component of the various types.

It is crucial to determine which type predominates. This is because such a determination guides treatment. Unless the dominant type is determined precise treatment is impossible to achieve. This is why the system of endocrine typing is so critical. Without it, the cause behind a condition may be completely missed.

Wrong treatment leads to poor results. This could prove disastrous. For instance, a person sees their doctor with fatigue, headaches, and depression, classic symptoms of sluggish thyroid. The doctor does tests and measures a slightly low-normal thyroid, while failing to evaluate adrenal status, which is, in fact, difficult to assess through blood testing. Assuming the problem is exclusively thyroid prescription hormone therapy is initiated. After taking the drug the patient becomes tense, hot, agitated, nervous, and weak. Then, pain develops, in the mid- to lower-back region. Quickly, the patient becomes exhausted and the depression deepens. He/she returns to the doctor and requests further evaluation.

The doctor fails to find anything further and, thus, prescribes antidepressants. Additional inspection reveals a low blood sodium, plus when the doctor examines the patient, he finds the pain in the mid- to lower-back to be severe. He orders x-rays, which are negative. This problem is, then, mis-diagnosed, perhaps as back strain, kidney trouble, or even anxiety. The doctor was unaware of the role of the adrenal glands and, thus, failed to determine the main cause of the symptoms, which is adrenal exhaustion. Surely, he/she didn't know how to type the body to determine which endocrine glands are involved.

By giving a potent drug, that is thyroid hormone, which activates the nervous system, the physician aggravated a dilemma. While he failed to realize it, the low sodium was of greater importance than the moderately low thyroid levels. It is an absolute marker of adrenal exhaustion. The doctor worsened the patient's endocrine imbalance by failing to make the correct diagnosis and by having no clue regarding the real cause of the symptoms. The patient is a combination type. Thus, all this could have been prevented by making a more accurate diagnosis and treating the adrenals as an additional focus.

Thyroid-adrenal types tend to be of medium height. Women with this type may tend towards modest weight gain, the fat being located in the lower front of the abdomen and along the hips. They can be thin but are usually somewhat overweight. They may hold some extra weight in the buttocks, in other words, they are not as flat in this region as pure thyroid types. Men may hold some extra weight in the front of the abdomen. Their hair is usually medium to medium-coarse. They do suffer tiredness and may find themselves falling asleep while at work during the day. There are often problems with concentration.

The main distinction is in the hands. Here, there is usually a combination of what is seen with the thyroid and adrenal types. On one hand the index finger is shorter than the ring finger (see Figure 8A right hand), and on the other hand the opposite is usually true (see Figure 8A left hand). In other words, the index finger is nearly as long or even longer than the ring finger. Thus, if on the dominant hand the index finger is shorter than the ring finger, this is thyroid-adrenal. However, if the opposite is true, that is on the dominant hand the index finger is longer than the ring finger, then, this is adrenal-thyroid (see Figure 8B).

Concentrate on the hand sign and the symptoms to determine if you are this type. Be sure to take both the thyroid and adrenal self tests, and compare the results. Those who score high on both tests most likely are combination types.

The diet for thyroid-adrenal is primarily the thyroid type, with, perhaps, the inclusion of modest amounts of complex carbohydrates. However, all refined starches and carbohydrates must be strictly avoided.

The body confirmation is a combination of the thyroid and adrenal types (study both diagrams).

Adrenal-thyroid type

In this type there is a reversal of the hand sign seen in the thyroid-adrenal type. Here, on the dominant hand the adrenal sign predominates. For instance, if a person is right-handed, the index finger is longer than the ring or about equal with the ring, whereas on the opposite hand the thyroid sign, that is a short index finger compared to the ring, predominates (see Figures 8A and 8B). Another variation of this type is where both index fingers are nearly as long as the ring fingers. Usually, with this type there is a higher score on the adrenal self-test than on the thyroid test.

The diet should be a combination of the foods recommended for adrenal and thyroid types. Coffee, tea, and chocolate should be avoided as well as white flour, commercial bread, and white rice. In particular, refined sugar must be strictly avoided. Usually, individuals with this type are intolerant to alcohol. Supplements for this type include undiluted 3x royal jelly, wild sage, wild rosemary, natural-source vitamin C, B complex, wild remote-source kelp, raw purple maca, and oregano juice. Unrefined salt should be used liberally in the diet.

Thyroid-muscular type (medium metabolizer, also known as muscular-pancreatic)

The muscular-thyroid type is usually medium in height. The neck is generally short and muscular. Or, in the taller example it may be long and muscular. The head tends to be rectangular. This type is often of medium height and stocky but not fat. Rarely, is such a person super-thin. This is the type of person, who is naturally well built.

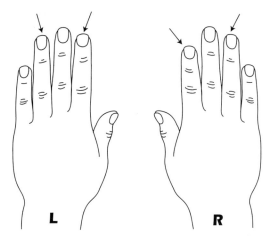

FIG. 8A Thyroid-adrenal hands, right hand dominant

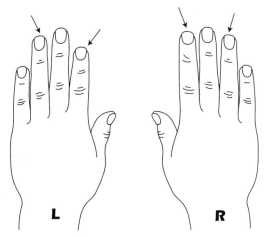

FIG. 8B Adrenal-thyroid hands, right hand dominant

Even so, often, as the person ages and also reduces activity he/she gains weight. Thus, in the later years the muscular type can maintain his or her physique only by keeping fit and watching the diet. These individuals are powerfully developed, particularly in their digestive organs, muscles, bones, and joints. They are usually strong but also agile.

In this type the muscles are noticeable, even if the person fails to work out. They just are naturally well built and strong. Their bodies are dramatically enhanced by training. While other types, such as certain pituitary and adrenal types, fail to tolerate exercise and are usually poorly muscled, the muscular-thyroid type desires exercise, in fact, thrives upon it. E. Benedict in her book *The Five Human Types* notes that this type is naturally "well upholstered" with firm muscles, while other people seem to be mere skin and bones or fat.

Thus, the muscular-thyroid type is the natural "he-man." Women can be muscular-thyroid. These are the women with broad shoulders and well-muscled hips and thighs. Yet, of course, in women this type is relatively rare. This is because women naturally have a special layer of fat plus a special delicate figure. In fact, naturally, women are soft, while men have a more firm structure.

Usually, the muscular-thyroid have square shoulders as well as a square chest. The thoracic cage is usually bulky, needed for providing oxygen to their massive muscles. It can also be long and muscular. They have enormous lung capacity, which facilitates their athletic prowess. The personality of such a person is usually just as powerful as their physique. Because of their efficient use of oxygen they rarely get sick. They are difficult to overpower and rarely suggestible. When they make up their minds about an issue, it is impossible to dissuade them. If there was a need for a powerful man, either in business or sports, this is the type of person that would be desired on the team.

The muscular-thyroid is vulnerable to weight gain. If such people neglect exercise, they readily gain weight. This is largely because they have a vigorous appetite, which is rarely manageable. They often eat huge quantities of food, largely to meet the needs of their muscular or strong frames.

Muscular types may vary in their build based upon their level of endocrine gland activity. If the pituitary gland is over-active, they may be short and stocky but usually are not grossly obese. They are big-boned or medium-boned and may be tall but usually are of average height or even short in stature. Their hands are often thick or big. The short stocky "coach" with big calves is the typical thyroid-muscular type.

The oxygen demands on this type are immense. Thus, even with all the exercise they may be oxygen-deficient. One way to check this is to look at the moons or lack thereof on the fingernails. Normally, on the first three fingers there should be a reasonably visible semi-circle. In this type the size of the moons on these fingers is smaller and in some cases non-existent. This is a sign of reduced oxygen metabolism in the body, a consequence of sluggish thyroid activity. This is why people with this type must exercise regularly. The size of the moons can be boosted through feeding the thyroid with the appropriate supplements which boost thyroid activity. This includes crude whole food northern Pacific kelp capsules, combined with wild rosemary herb. The crushed wild oregano in capsule and powder form is also therapeutic, as is the juice or hydrosol of wild oregano. Wild rosemary juice/essence also boosts blood flow to the thyroid and the rest of the body, while increasing the capacity of the cells to use oxygen. So does wild rosemary oil. The intake of seafood would also be medicinal, since this provides the thyroid with much needed salts, particularly the salts of iodine, bromine, and chloride. Natural wild riboflavin, as found in wild greens flush, also helps oxygenate the tissues. So does the consumption of organic red meat.

This type is also known as muscular-pancreatic. This is because the pancreas is another dominant organ for these individuals. They need powerful pancreatic activity for protein digestion, that is to supply the great needs of their muscles for amino acids. So, here, digestive enzymes are a key supplement. Thyroid-muscular types should regularly take digestive enzymes.

The pituitary-thyroid-adrenal type

This is the most rare and serious of all endocrine types. In this case all the endocrine glands are dysfunctional. These people have features common to all three main types. This is demonstrated by the fact that they score significantly on all written tests. The body shape of this type has features mainly of the pituitary type with a tendency for increased abdominal fat or even swelling. The finger length varies, but the hands are usually short and stubby. The fingers are often swollen.

The simple way to know if a person has this type is to take the tests and see if there is a reasonably high score in all three categories. Also, see if the hands are this configuration, that is rather short with swollen fingers. Often, the index finger and ring finger are nearly the same length, although, occasionally, the index finger is slightly longer than the ring. The head is more round than square. The hair is medium to medium-fine. There is usually a fat pad about the lateral ankle. There is also a drooping of fat or tissue from the first part of the triceps. The shoulders may be hunched with fat pads. People with this type usually have poor energy and often crave sweets and chocolate.

These people have significant endocrine imbalances to such a degree that they are often diseased. It is in this type that serious endocrine disorders are most common such as polycystic ovarian disease, endometriosis, infertility, impotence, pituitary tumor, menorrhagia (excessive menstruation), and amenorrhea (lack of menstruation). Also, people with this type may suffer from hirsutism, which is male pattern hair in females. Treatment is to follow largely the pituitary diet, with the modification of an increase in salt intake. As well, supplements must be aggressively taken. The supplements for pituitary and adrenal types should be combined.

People with weak pituitary glands always have weak adrenal glands. This is a type of syndrome, where the adrenal component can be more significant than the pituitary one. In this case the adrenal weakness is the focus. Boosting adrenal function, in fact, balances the pituitary. So does boosting thyroid function. The typical allergic individual, the one who readily reacts to chemicals in foods, is this type. This is especially true if such a person develops head or brain-related symptoms. Reactions to foods can be severe and may include dizziness, fainting, migraine headaches, and even seizures. The person with epilepsy may have this.

Since this type is the most complex some of the features must be reiterated. Usually, people with this type are of medium height or short. They may tend, like adrenal types, to have a long index finger on one hand, or both index fingers are as long or a bit longer than the ring fingers. Abdominally, there is often a pouch typically from the umbilicus down, in other words, usually, they are plump. Or, they have a beach ball abdomen. The point is these people are usually rotund.

Sensitivity to smells is high, as is sensitivity to touch and noise. The skin is also sensitive, and there may be blemishes. These people are generally tired and require much sleep.

The shape of the hips is distinctive. In women, in particular there is a fair amount of weight from about the mid-upper thigh downward. This is a sign of ovarian dysfunction. The shoulders are small and slope downward. However, in contrast to the true pituitary type the head is usually normal size for the body.

Pituitary types: vulnerabilities

The main feature is extreme sensitivity. Typically, this is the person who must follow a restrictive diet, because of intense food allergy reactions. Plus, again, such a person is highly sensitive to fumes and toxic chemicals. These are the individuals who react so severely to noxious odors that they seem to know before anyone else if there is a poisonous substance in the air. Thus, they have a high sensitivity to smells, especially from noxious substances.

People with pituitary components are easily poisoned by chemicals in their food and/or water. Toxicity can result both from natural and synthetic chemicals. Toxic chemicals are highly disruptive to the glands, especially the pituitary and adrenals. Synthetic chemicals which cause such disruption include herbicides, pesticides, solvents, fungicides, and various synthetic food additives.

One of the most toxic of all poisons are the fungal toxins, known as mycotoxins. These naturally occurring toxins are even more poisonous than many synthetic chemicals in terms of the mass disruption they cause in the body. Mycotoxins are particularly disruptive to the endocrine glands. These are poisons made by the fungi themselves, including those that reside in the human body. These fungal poisons greatly disrupt metabolism. Rapidly, they corrupt endocrine function, usually causing massive inflammation in these organs. Mycotoxins have a special predilection for the pituitary and adrenal glands, which they readily poison.

The endocrine glands are highly vulnerable to such poisons, because of their high rate of metabolism. Thus, again, for the majority of people with significant endocrine disorders commercial grains, as well as peanut butter and corn, must be avoided. This is largely because of the mycotoxin content of such foods.

Even so, regarding grains they are nutritionally poor. This is evident from any food chart. It will be discovered that, for instance, corn, rye, and wheat are relatively low in nutrients. Certainly, such foods are nutritionally inferior to the various foods recommended in this book. Plus, rye and wheat are difficult to digest, far more so than, for instance, meat or poultry. The exception is peanut butter. It is, in fact, highly nutritionally dense, since it is a rich source of protein as well as vitamins. It is also readily digested. In particular, it is an excellent source of niacin, riboflavin, pantothenic acid, and thiamine. It may be eaten, but only if it is decontaminated. To achieve this add spice oils into it, and then, mix. This will neutralize the mycotoxins.

One such spice oil, which is ideal for this purpose, is oil of wild oregano. Simply mix 10 drops of the wild hand-picked emulsified oil in an extra virgin olive oil base in eight ounces of peanut butter. Then, it can be safely eaten. Even so, peanut butter should be eaten in moderation.

People with pituitary weakness may be allergic to peanuts and peanut butter. Some people are so allergic to peanut butter that even if it is decontaminated, they react. Thus, for such individuals it should be completely avoided. For this body type, in fact, nuts and nut butters are preferable, the best nut butters being those made from filberts, macadamias, almonds, and pumpkin seeds. People with adrenal weakness may also be allergic to peanuts and other legumes but may eat nuts freely.

There are other reasons for avoiding grains. Since they are high in starch they also may feed fungal growth. Plus, commercial grains contain bizarre anti-hormone substances known as lectins. These substances are highly toxic to the pituitary.

This may explain a significant dilemma. For instance, in societies where grains are the staple short stature, that is growth retardation, is common. In certain parts of Iran, where wheat is the main source of calories, stunted growth is the norm. This may be due to the fact that wheat destroys critical growth factors, such as the hormones, as well as certain growth inducing nutrients such as zinc and vitamin A. Zinc is readily destroyed by wheat and to a lesser degree rye. Yet, this mineral is essential for normal bone, muscular, and organ development.

Wheat is a relative of the grasses. It provides only minimal nourishment and, certainly, fails to sustain vital health. Wheat germ, which contains certain hormones, might be an exception. However, due to the frequency of wheat allergy the germ may act as a toxin, aggravating health problems or even causing ill health.

Alternative grains may be well tolerated. Such grains include kamut and spelt. Yet, these are wheat derivatives, and thus, those who are sensitive to wheat must avoid them. Whole oats may be tolerated. Brown rice is low in mycotoxins and, thus, can be incorporated into this program. Amaranth, quinoa, and teff are also acceptable. For anyone with pituitary weakness the key is to avoid toxic reactions, especially to legumes. This is why the diet is restrictive. Only through a toxin-free diet can the person with disabled or weakened glands expect to rapidly heal.

It is a great deal of work to find such grains and grain flours. It is additional work to bake one's own foods. However, since the result is superior health it is well worth the effort. Thus, for those who must have grains, an effort must be made to find alternative flours, and bake your own products.

Grain products pre-made with such flours may be available. Look for breads made with rice or millet flour, which are less likely to be mold-contaminated. Regardless, the best grains are not even grains. They are instead seeds. Thus, flour made from brown rice, wild rice, millet, amaranth, quinoa, and teff are, metabolically, ideal.

Commercial grains are contaminated with mold toxins, largely because of the way they are stored. It is difficult to prevent mold growth during such storage. Or, the grain may be contaminated in the field, especially if it is over-wintered. Also, these grains are hybrids, so their immune systems are weak, and they are readily attacked by molds. Such toxicity can be prevented simply by avoiding the primary commercial grains, which are vulnerable to mold contamination. These are wheat, rye, corn, and barley. Oats are less vulnerable, so as a last resort this may be consumed.

Regarding this the ideal type is oat bran. This may be purchased for making a hot cereal. Oat bran is relatively low in carbohydrates, and for those who tolerate it this grain makes an ideal addition to the breakfast menu. Simply follow directions and cook, but try not to cook it excessively. Top with a pat or two of butter along with half and half or whole milk; add cinnamon and/or cloves for taste. A major reason to always add these spices is that they aid in carbohydrate metabolism. In particular, cinnamon acts as a natural insulin, in fact, reducing the insulin surge. Thus, when eating starchy cereals, be liberal with the cinnamon.

For an even more powerful taste, as well as action, use the edible oil of cinnamon in an extra virgin olive oil base (blue label). It is a CO_2 (super critical) extract, which is rich in flavonoids. Through the use of CO_2 extraction the full power of the flavonoids is preserved. Because these flavonoids are unaltered they impart an unusually rich flavor. Only a few drops flavors any dish.

Chapter Six

Strengthening Your
Hormone System

The body needs nutrients for survival. All cells require key nutrients for their function, longevity, and repair. Eating for the hormone type means to supply the nutrients which assist the function of the glands and which even preserve these glands. Certain nutrients are crucial for normal metabolism. These nutrients are needed for all glands and include the vitamins, minerals, fatty acids, sterols (and steroids), tissue salts, and amino acids/proteins. The following section focuses on such nutrients. Yet, in particular the glands have a high need for fatty substances, including fat soluble vitamins and cholesterol. The majority of hormones are derived from cholesterol, which is a lipid. So, this section will focus on fatty nutrients as well as other key nutrients.

Fat soluble vitamins: the glands' saviors

It was the dentist Weston Price who first recognized the critical importance of fat soluble vitamins for glandular

189

health. He determined that the health of the endocrine system was in top condition in people whose diets were rich in these vitamins. He wrote an entire book on how native diets rich in natural fats and fatty nutrients greatly strengthened body function. This was largely through the creation of powerful glandular reserves. Essentially, the diets were rich in fatty hormones and their precursors.

People who violate this function through eating commercial and processed foods suffer from exhausted glands. Also, those who eat only vegetation violate this and thus suffer the consequences. These consequences are exhaustion, muscular weakness, bone loss, muscle atrophy, weakness of the heart, and, ultimately, brain/nerve damage. This is because animal sources of cholesterol and its derivatives, as well as animal-source hormones, are essential for the proper function and structure of these systems.

This explains the exhaustion suffered by such people, that is those who subsist only on vegetation. This is not an attempt to criticize those who follow such a diet. Rather, it is merely an analysis of who vegetation-only diets impact physiology. Price was able to prove that poor diet, that is diet lacking key endocrine factors, such as animal-source cholesterol, vitamin A, and vitamin D, directly damages the endocrine tissues, while a completely natural diet, which includes raw foods, preserved function. This derogatory diet affects both the physical appearance and the sense of wellness. The generations gradually become weakened. Ultimately, this leads to the destruction of civilization.

People who were strong and fit consumed the critical fatty components. These components were dubbed by Price as "factor X." Those who did not consume them became physically weak. Their physiques became deformed. They were simply lacking those hormones and pre-hormones needed for vital growth. This precisely explains the dilemma of Western humans, whose diets are grossly deficient in this factor.

Fat soluble vitamins promote strength. These vitamins are needed to produce hormones. Can anyone think of a creature more powerful than a polar bear? It thrives upon factor X. The polar bear flourishes in the most hostile climate known, all by consuming a greater amount of these factors than any other creature. Without these factors polar bears degenerate and ultimately die.

The fat soluble vitamins, notably vitamins A and D, plus their analogues, are needed for a wide range of "strength"-related functions. Hormone synthesis is dependent upon them. These substances are critical for building and maintaining strong bones and joints. They help keep the teeth, as well as gums, strong. They are needed for bolstering immune function. They help keep the linings of the body, that is the mucous membranes, in top condition.

Vitamin A is one of the most critical components of the fat soluble factors. It is essential for the development and growth of all mucous membranes. In this regard it is essential for the synthesis of the highly protective secretory IgA, which is the immune system's front line defense against infections, toxicity, and allergy. This secretory factor is secreted directly along the mucous linings, a process dependent upon vitamin A. Food is the ideal source of this vitamin. Top sources are fatty foods such as butter, egg yolk, fatty fish, whole milk products, and organ meats. Only animal foods contain it.

Vitamins A and D are essential for growth. If they are lacking, stunting of growth will occur. All cells need these vitamins, both for reproduction and overall health. In particular, all the linings of the body, the so-called body tracts, require vitamin A. These linings are constantly exposed to toxins as well as germs. If this vitamin is lacking, the linings degenerate, making them vulnerable to infection and disease. Once they degenerate the cells of these linings are no longer able to process toxins. The cellular lining, normally a key barrier against germs, becomes so weak that germs readily penetrate it. The tissue linings are an enormously valuable defense. They fully block invasion by germs. They act to trap toxins, as well as foreign materials, not only germs but also particles, which can act as irritants. Thus, strong healthy tissue linings are the ideal defense against virtually all diseases, even cancer.

Strong and healthy cells, which line the tissues, known as epithelial cells, are an effective means for preventing illness, infection, and even serious disease. Vitamin A, as well as vitamin D, control the synthesis of such cells. To protect the body against cancer, heart disease, arthritis, digestive disorders, and similar degenerative conditions it is necessary to regularly include vitamin A- and D-rich foods in the diet. Top sources include liver, kidney, whole milk products, butter, cheese, yogurt, egg yolk, and fatty fish, fish liver oil, and the fatty skin of animals. Again, there are no vegetable sources of these vitamins. Therefore, vegetarians and, particularly, vegans are grossly deficient in these key nutrients. This can wreak havoc on the mucous membranes as well as the gums, bones, and teeth.

To a degree this can be compensated for by the regular intake of crude undiluted royal jelly. Here, a 3x royal jelly and/or royal jelly paste emulsified in crude cold-pressed pumpkinseed oil is invaluable. Also, if possible, a small dose of cod liver oil should be taken, like a teaspoon daily. Ideally, this should be taken in a heavy fat such as butter, crude cold-pressed sesame oil, or extra virgin olive oil. Such supplements can help ward off serious diseases due to vitamin A and/or D deficiency such as pneumonia, growth retardation, thyroid cysts/tumors, stomach atrophy, hypochlorhydria (low or absent stomach acid), heart disease, osteoporosis, and cancer. Also, the lack of these fat soluble vitamins may explain the fact that sudden fractures are ultra–common in strict vegans.

It is realized that there is a hesitancy to eat certain foods due to contamination. Yet, the body requires certain nutrients found only in animal sources. For instance, liver is the ideal source of fat soluble vitamins. However, since the liver concentrates toxins, this is not always desirable. Thus, the only recommended source is organic liver or, perhaps, fish liver oils. Of course, fish liver oils are the most concentrated source, far more so than animal liver. Thus, cod liver oil and halibut liver oil serve as invaluable sources of these factors. Herring and sardine oils are also excellent sources, since such tiny fish concentrate less toxins than larger fish. However, by far the ideal source is wild Alaskan sockeye salmon oil. This is because this is the least refined of all fish-based vitamin A and D sources. It is also because studies show that of all fish sockeye salmon are the lowest in contaminants, including mercury.

Fish eggs, that is roe, is yet another source. The body stores few vitamins. Vitamins A and D are among the few it aggressively stores. B_{12} is another such vitamin. The question must be asked, why does the body focus on storing these nutrients? It becomes obvious that these vitamins are critical to the survival of the organism. Without them, the tissues degenerate and disease readily strikes.

The sources of such regenerative substances in the human diet are few, these substances with so-called factor X activity. A rather complete list of factor X-rich foods and supplements includes:

- whole organic butter
- whole organic cream
- whole organic milk
- organic liver (or other organ meats)
- fish roe
- fatty fish
- unprocessed royal jelly (ideally fortified with wild sage and rosemary, which boost the action of the naturally occurring factor X compounds)
- bee pollen and raw honey
- fish liver oil
- crude unprocessed pumpkinseed oil
- unprocessed, raw maca extract (liquid form)
- crude steam extracted wild-source sockeye salmon oil (available as pinkish-colored oil in an 8-ounce bottle and fish gelatin capsules)

The importance of fatty compounds

People have a distorted idea of about fats. There are those who are even paranoid about this. They think that, somehow, fat—that is the natural fats in foods—could harm or even kill them. Yet, such fats are essential parts of the diet and can cause no significant harm.

Even so, the misconceptions abound. For instance, just because a person is overweight doesn't mean that the person must avoid fat. Yet, such a one could be overweight because of a deficiency of fat. This is because weight problems are largely deficiency diseases, and deficiencies direly affect the endocrine glands. Thus, there are certain fats or fat soluble nutrients which, if lacking, cause obesity. What is true is that there are certain fats which are good or healthy fats, while there are others which are bad or harmful. This means that certain fats may be eaten freely without concern, that is as a source of key nutrients. In fact, the consumption of these fats must be greatly encouraged. On the contrary, there are certain fats, which due to their harsh or toxic effects upon the body, must be strictly avoided. In contrast, the safety of pure natural fats is beyond dispute. The dangerous ones are the synthetic or heavily processed fats such as hydrogenated oils, partially hydrogenated oils, lard, cottonseed oil, and refined vegetable oils.

This immense value of naturally occurring fats, including saturated fats, was discovered decades ago by medical researchers. As mentioned previously it largely began with work by a dentist, Westin Price, who found that in societies where natural or saturated fats were eaten freely various diseases common to the civilized peoples were unknown. He found that the primitives who regularly ate these fats were free of dental diseases, that is tooth decay, tooth malformation, and gum diseases, as well as heart disease, hardening of the arteries, cancer, and arthritis. In the 1930s fascinating work at the University of Wisconsin confirmed this. By accident researchers noted that the natural fats in milk, in this case, butter, stimulated growth better than the feeding of skim milk alone. In other words, the fat contained certain nutrients required for cellular growth.

These researchers also found that the animal fat helped cellular health more superiorly than vegetable fats such as corn and coconut oils. This is a critical finding, that animal fat is a cell- and organ-building substance, while many vegetable oils do not offer this property. Their conclusion was that the saturated fats of animal origin, specifically the natural fats of milk, contain growth factors, which are necessary for human development.

These researchers were far from promoting an industry. They were merely making the observation that there are substances in concentrated animal fats which are essential to human nutrition and which are impossible to supply through vegetation. In further research by Price published in the *American Journal of Public Health* it was clearly shown that the vital health of animals and, therefore, humans is dependent upon animal-source fats. In rats the feeding of mere vegetable oils alone led to poor development of the body, in fact, growth was stunted. Even if cod liver oil was added to the feed, the growth was relatively poor. When animal-source fats, in this case vitamin concentrates from butter, were added to the rations, growth of all systems, particularly the bones and joints, was spurred. Thus, the animal fats provide the missing link: factor X. This is how almighty God made it. He made the herbivore for the sake of humankind as a means to concentrate nutrients.

Growth is evidence of true vitality: of life itself. It is the marker of a being's power. Think about a poorly formed child versus a well formed one. Actually, growth, bone density, and dentition are signs of vitality, of superior health.

A weak feeble person is disregarded, perhaps abused. A powerful full-boned person is admired, even feared. Yet, in fact, Price found that the more well nourished a person was the more calm and less violent he was. There was a serene nature of the natural fat eaters, which was obvious.

The powerful effects of saturated fats are largely due to the fatty vitamins. However, there are also hormonal factors in such food with immense powers. Price mentions the case of a child with a broken leg. The child also had seizures. The leg failed to heal, and the child was overall weak and nervous. By the mere addition of milk fat to the diet in the form of whole milk and a butter concentrate not only did the fracture heal but also the nervousness, weakness, and seizures were cured. Price attributed the cure primarily to the intake of butter. He used a special type of butter, which was high in vitamins. Within a month the non-healing fracture was cured and the cast removed. X-rays proved that there was a remarkable improvement, with complete healing and a high bone deposition. Thus, the entire mineral metabolism of this three-year-old was normalized by the animal concentrates. Said Price, "a non-closing fracture of six months' standing made a marked improvement in 35 days."

This kind of healing would today be regarded as a miracle, yet few if any doctors would consider a whole milk and butter feed curative for such a lesion. This is despite the fact that it has been proven that the consumption of unprocessed whole milk products, even butter, stimulate both calcium absorption and also deposition into bone. Price demonstrated this in his case. He measured the blood calcium levels as well as phosphorus and magnesium levels. All levels rose dramatically on the whole milk-butter therapy. Also, raw whole milk contains key minerals needed by all cells in the body, including tissue salts.

Yet, today, physicians fail to recommend the consumption of such foods for reversing bone injuries. This is demonstrated by a more recent case, the famous basketball player, Bill Walton. He had no capacity to build bone, because he lacked the essential activating factors, notably vitamins A and D. Bill Walton, an enormous man with thick bones, had a promising career in professional basketball. However, he fractured his ankle, and it failed to heal. Later, it was discovered that he was a strict vegan, which compromised his nutritional status. Walton lost his entire career due to a faulty diet.

Even so, obviously, today commercial milk is inadequate as a healing agent. This is largely due to the excessive use of chemicals, including the genetically engineered bovine growth hormone as well as antibiotics. Here, raw organic milk would be ideal for healing and curing disease. If such milk is available, a few drops of oil of wild oregano and oil of cinnamon bark (emulsified in extra virgin olive oil) per liter ensure Sterility.

Pesticides are used on cattle, residues of which are absorbed into the milk. This neutralizes any healing attributes. However, truly organic milk, even if it is homogenized and pasteurized, can provide some of these benefits. Even so, it's best to get the unhomogenized type. Thus, in the event of bone damage, fractures, tooth decay, and/or gum disease the regular intake of a high quality organic butter and/or organic whole milk is advised. Such foods are also advisable in the event of growth failure in children. Price went further with his research to prove their importance. In this regard he found that in all people who ate fresh or raw milk, bone and dental disease were unknown.

There has been much propaganda, largely promoted by the vegetarian and vegan movements, that milk is poisonous for humans. The oft-repeated adage, "Milk is only for baby cows" has influenced virtually everyone. This is perhaps true of commercial milk: these issues aren't being contested. Some people are direly allergic to it and must strictly avoid it. Even so, what is clear is that there are critical nutritional factors in milk which are impossible to derive from vegetation. Besides, cows and other animals process vegetable matter into highly condensed human food, which is milk and, ultimately, yogurt and cheese. These foods are true nutrient concentrates, which are readily digested. What's more, people are vulnerable to a deficiency of such animal source nutrients, notably calcium, phosphorus, magnesium, taurine, carotene, pantothenic acid, riboflavin, vitamin B_{12}, vitamin A, and vitamin D. None of such nutrients can be readily obtained in grains, vegetables, or fruit. Even so, the level of such nutrients gradually declines in virtually all people after the teenage years. Thus, for ideal health a vigorous effort should be made to replenish tissue stores of these nutrients.

Unless these nutrients are regularly replaced a chronic deficiency must occur. Here, Price clearly proved that the incorporation of rather modest amounts of milk and milk concentrates, when combined with healthy mineral-rich food, dramatically improve nutritional status, that is by causing a definite measurable increase in the blood of key nutrients, notably calcium, phosphorus, magnesium, and, of course, vitamins A and D. The latter vitamins are critical growth factors for the skeletal system.

B$_{12}$: the meaty nutrient

It is not only milk products which contain critical growth factors, but these growth factors are also found in meat. Actually, meat contains certain factors difficult to procure in milk products, notably intrinsic factor, vitamin B$_{12}$, tissue salts, carnitine, tissue hormones, and folic acid. All these factors are essential for the growth and health of the tissues.

Growth is important for all ages. This is because the body is constantly reproducing cells: billions of them daily. Unless the body is supplied with sufficient supplies of growth factors, cells and organs will develop abnormally. Bizarre growths will occur. This is because the cells develop into freakish forms in the absence of growth factors. This may ultimately lead to degenerative diseases. Thus, to be in optimal health the body must be routinely supplied with the key growth factors necessary for maintaining the health of all cells and organs. These factors are found primarily in foods of animal origin. Animals require such growth factors. That is why they are so powerful and dense. Plants rely upon the sun for growth. Animals rely primarily upon plant food as the source of their power.

Vitamin B$_{12}$ is a key nutrient found only in animal foods. This vitamin is one of the most potent cell growth factors known. In humans it is necessary for the growth of all tissues, especially the nervous system. Seaweed contains a miniscule amount, but this is largely because it is contaminated with bacteria and other animal wastes. What's more, the form of B$_{12}$ in seaweed is poorly utilized compared to the animal type. Only animals synthesize this vitamin. Maca root is perhaps the only significant land vegetable source of this nutrient.

B_{12} is a critical vitamin. Without it, the body is vulnerable to severe damage. The greatest damage is suffered by the central nervous system, that is the brain and spinal cord. Here, the damage can be permanent. Signs and symptoms of B_{12} deficiency are primarily neurological and include depression, agitation, irritability, numbness/tingling, loss of sensation, memory loss, shock-like sensations, acute and severe eye pain/headaches, and a sensation where the feet feel too big for the shoes. There may also be numbness in the bottom of the feet. Burning tongue is another warning sign, and in the extreme the tongue becomes beet red, which is known as magenta tongue. It may also become enlarged and swollen, which is known as macroglossia. Anorexia may occur, since B_{12} is needed for normal stomach function.

The reason a deficiency of this nutrient is so devastating for the nervous system is that B_{12} is needed for nerve cell regeneration. Without it, nerve cells die. Plus, it is an essential cofactor in the production of critical brain chemicals such as serotonin, dopamine, and norepinephrine. The latter substances, known as neurotransmitters, are essential for the function of all brain, spinal cord, and nerve cells.

It has been long known that a prolonged deficiency of this vitamin results in dire consequences. This is because the deficiency causes a condition known as *sub-acute combined degeneration*. This term itself is somewhat descriptive. It is manifested by what appears to be a sudden loss in neurological function due to inflammation of the brain and spinal cord. Yet, it is far from sudden. The degeneration occurs systematically over months or years, although the extreme symptoms may develop suddenly, which include an ALS(Lou Gehrig's)-like presentation involving loss of muscle and nerve control. However, the 'acute' phase occurs only once the damage becomes extreme, manifested largely by a stripping of the normal fatty coating of the nerves, a process known as demyelination. This is because B_{12} facilitates the building up of the insulation around the nerve sheaths.

Without this nutrient the production and/or repair of the insulation stalls. Once the nerves lose their highly protective insulation various symptoms develop, plus the nerves become exceptionally vulnerable to infection, since the insulation is a barrier against germs. Demyelination occurs in a variety of diseases, including multiple sclerosis, Parkinson's disease, dementia, Alzheimer's, and ALS. It is also common in people on restrictive diets, particularly vegans. Additionally, the elderly due to poor food preparation, inability to chew, and disease may develop such syndromes. This is because of both a dietary lack of the vitamin as well as poor absorption. Regarding absorption it is a lack of hydrochloric acid which is the key factor, since this acid is needed to break apart B_{12} from food.

Virtually all neurological diseases appear to be tied to B_{12} deficiency. As described in *Life Extension* magazine reduced levels have been measured in patients with Alzheimer's disease, and the vitamin may help reverse some of the symptoms of seemingly incurable diseases such as ALS, dementia, Parkinson's disease, Alzheimer's disease, and multiple sclerosis. What's more, in certain types of depression and anxiety B_{12} deficiency is a primary causative factor. Psychosis may also be related to the deficiency.

Again, B_{12} is virtually exclusively an animal-derived vitamin found mainly in herbivores. With their complex digestive systems, animals or, rather, microbes in the gut of such animals synthesize it from various hydrocarbons. Thus, it is bacterial fermentation in the abdomen of cattle which is the real source of this vitamin. This is why meat and particularly organ meats are rich sources. This is in sufficient quantities to prevent deficiency if meat products, along with organ meats, are regularly consumed. In contrast, there are no significant vegetable sources of this vitamin. This is why according to *Life Extension* vegans and strict vegetarians "are at risk for B_{12} deficiency."

Yet, eating meat and other top sources may fail to correct the deficiency. This is because many individuals poorly absorb this vitamin. This is largely due to a deficiency of key factors needed for its absorption, mainly stomach acid and intrinsic factor. Both these substances are produced within the stomach wall.

In certain individuals there is an acquired or inherited tendency to fail to produce sufficient quantities of these factors. This is known as pernicious anemia. It may also be called autoimmune disease of the stomach. Here, the stomach fails to produce sufficient secretions in order to facilitate absorption. The vitamin is held tightly within animal protein. Acid is needed to release it from these bonds, and the intrinsic factor is needed to bind to this vitamin, so it can be transported into the blood. Disorders of the stomach commonly lead to a reduction in stomach acid production. Also, the B_{12}, once bound to intrinsic factor, is transported into the blood through the membranes of the lower small intestine. Inflammation of the small intestine also disrupts absorption. So, it becomes obvious how disease of the gut can lead to deficiency.

The greatest dilemma is the inadequate production of stomach acid. This condition may be caused by chronic infection, which destroys the lining of the stomach. The failure to produce sufficient intrinsic factor may also be due to infection. Surely, H. pylori plays a role in this damage. However, there are, perhaps, numerous yet-to-be determined germs, including fungi, which disrupt stomach acid production.

Again, vitamin B_{12} is by far the largest known vitamin. Thus, the body has difficulty with its absorption. Without stomach acid and/or intrinsic factor it is virtually impossible to absorb. There are other factors which affect absorption. Antacids and H-2 blocking drugs, such as Tagamet, Zantac, Prilosec, Pepcid, Nexium, and similar agents, greatly obstruct B_{12} absorption. Such drugs should never be consumed, since they greatly disrupt the normal physiology. Cortisone and certain antibiotics may also interfere with its absorption. Gastric stapling or bypass devastate it. People who receive this operation are a great risk for deficiency. Such individuals must routinely take B_{12} supplements.

Alcohol also destroys this nutrient, plus it greatly interferes with its absorption. Alcohol destroys the stomach lining, which eventually results in a life-threatening B_{12} deficiency. This is because the stomach makes intrinsic factor, the critical substance needed for B_{12} absorption. With chronic alcohol consumption there is extensive damage to the stomach wall, a condition known as atrophic gastritis. It is also known as alcoholic gastritis. In such a condition intrinsic factor is no longer produced, and, therefore, B_{12} deficiency develops.

Cholesterol: key to hormonal health

The importance of cholesterol as a critical nutrient has been underestimated. In fact, this nutrient is one of the most crucial of all dietary substances. An effort must be made to consume it on a regular basis, that is for ideal health. This is true for all hormone types. Yet, it is particularly true for those with the adrenal type, since cholesterol is the building block for the production of steroid hormones. It is also a key substance for those suffering from ovarian or testicular disorders. In this regard it is needed for the reversal of infertility.

Cholesterol makes an individual strong. It is a primary growth factor. Restricting it from the diet may lead to stunting of growth. It is the key substance for strengthening cell walls. For babies if it is restricted, there are many catastrophes. There is failure to thrive. There is a halting of growth. There is retardation. Ultimately, death occurs.

This wax is also the key agent for keeping the cells of the brain and spinal cord cells in top condition. The brain, as is signified by its yellow color, largely consists of cholesterol. Incredibly, diseases of the nervous system may be largely due to cholesterol deficiency.

Cholesterol is produced in vast quantities in the liver. This is because it is required by all cells in the body. So, the body produces it profusely, manufacturing it in the liver and to a lesser degree ovaries, testes, and adrenals. Surely, this demonstrates the critical nature of this substance. In fact, the equivalent of a dozen eggs worth of this wax is produced in the body on a daily basis.

Why does the body produce wax? It is because this wax is a cellular sealant. Plus, it is the key precursor to hormone synthesis. Therefore, arbitrarily forcing it out of the body can only lead to devastation. Actually, this wax is one of the body's most critical substances of the body. It is precisely this substance which is used to repair cellular damage to

206 The Body Shape Diet

prevent leakage of cell contents. It is also needed for making cell walls impervious to germs. Cholesterol is the primary agent for repairing cell wall damage, and this includes the walls of the arteries. Without it, the cells of the body are highly vulnerable to germ invasion, especially by viruses. It is also needed for digestion and absorption. The thorough digestion of fat is dependent upon this substance, that is through the production of bile. The latter is a fat emulsifier. Also, cholesterol is needed to make critical substances in the blood, known as HDL and LDL proteins. These are effective fat-transporting molecules, incredibly, the body uses a wax to transport fat.

Deficiency of cholesterol is serious. This happens frequently, especially with the constant effort of some individuals to reduce their cholesterol levels. Doctors have made cholesterol the enemy, especially for cardiovascular conditions. In fact, it wasn't the doctors who did this. This is a plot by the pharmaceutical industry to sell drugs. Yet, cholesterol plays no major role in heart disease. Rather, it protects against it. This is why the body produces it in such vast quantities. Since it is a wax it acts as a sealant within the blood vessels. In other words, the body uses it to heal damage, both within the blood vessels and heart as well as various other tissues. In fact, more heart attacks occur in people with low cholesterol levels than in those with moderately high levels. This is because these heart attack victims are deficient in this sealant. It is this sealant which prevents the weakening of the arterial walls. It even prevents the heart muscle from weakening.

There is another major reason why its lack leads to weakness. Cholesterol is the key substance for the production of the majority of the body's hormones.

Moreover, it is these hormones which are responsible for a person's strength and power. The body makes cholesterol constantly. In this regard it is more critical than mere vitamins. Why would anyone seek to force it out of the body? Nearly 100 different hormones within the body are made from it. This includes some 60 different adrenal steroids, several types of vitamin D, DHEA, estrogen, progesterone, and testosterone plus dozens of others. Without it, the hormone system fails. If it is supplied consistently, the endocrine system is empowered, resulting in enormous strength and excellent health.

The degree of ignorance within the medical profession is unfathomable. There is no proof that simply a rise in cholesterol levels causes heart disease nor that forcibly lowering it prevents it. Heart disease is due to poor diet. It is caused by excessive alcohol consumption. Stress also plays a major role. Gum disease plays a significant role. It is largely due to toxicity, for instance, toxic petrochemical or heavy metal poisoning. It is often the result of infections, for instance, infection of the arteries by herpes, nanobacter, candida, and/or chlamydia and the infection of the heart valves by strep or staph. So, a high cholesterol level may be a marker of stress or inflammation. To suddenly force this level down will upset body chemistry.

Forcibly lowering cholesterol might seemingly aid the heart. Yet, such an approach damages the various other organs, particularly the brain, muscles, kidneys, and spinal cord. This is a diabolic approach to supposed health improvement. It is clearly further evidence of the barbarism of modern medicine, that is that the cause is never treated, while only the symptoms are addressed. A high cholesterol level is merely a symptom of disordered metabolism as well as inappropriate diet. Thus, the metabolism must be corrected and the diet improved in order to reverse this.

The cholesterol should not be forcibly reduced, since a high level is not the cause of anything. It is only a reaction, signalling an imbalance in the body. For instance, consider cholesterol-lowering drugs. While the claim is that they reduce the incidence of heart disease they, in fact, heighten the incidence of a variety of other diseases. As demonstrated by a Finnish study published at the University of Helsinki regular use increases the risks for cancer 600%, while the risks for violent deaths, including suicide, rise some 300%. Moreover, there is no real value in such drugs, because even with the risk for heart disease there is no proof of any benefit. Why place the body at such risks when the facts refute the value? Even with heart disease the potential damage from a high or moderate level of cholesterol is far outweighed by the risk from the drugs. Plus, the risk for disease from a low level is far higher than a high one. In fact, levels below 160 are deadly.

Even so, for people with metabolic disorder and resulting high cholesterol levels there is a natural supplement, which safely reduces or rather normalizes levels. This is a combination of remote-grown cumin extract as well as wild northern Pacific kelp and red sour grape. Powerful, this complex routinely normalizes abnormal cholesterol levels.

God made fats. He included them in enormous amounts of foods. In natural forms they cause the body no harm. Rather, they are essential for proper nutrition and organ function. Stripping the fats out of the diet leads to disease, not good health. Why violate nature when all has been so perfectly designed? There is thorough proof that by corrupting natural fats or forcibly eliminating them from the diet only negative results occur. The body makes great use of the natural fats found in various healthy foods: the fat of milk, the lipids of eggs, the natural fat in beef or lamb, or the natural fats in nuts, seeds, olives, and avocados.

Has anyone 'died' from eating such foods? Is there any record of a person developing an illness or dying from eating, for instance, steak and eggs, avocados, handfuls of nuts, with the exception of nut (or legume in the case of peanuts) allergy, a few pats of butter, or some heavy cream? On the contrary, such foods have a history of helping peoples' health by providing nutrients in a natural and usable form. Price in his book *Physical Degeneration* proved that diets lacking such naturally occurring fatty foods led to outright degeneration of the tissues. Animal studies by Roger Williams, Ph.D., showed that when processed foods, stripped of their natural fats, are fed to test animals the animals become sick. Their arteries degenerate. Their coat of hair appears sickly, their bone structure is weakened, and their growth is stunted. If the missing fats, in this instance, milk fat, is replaced, the degenerative changes are reversed.

Omega-3 oils: critical cofactors

Everyone knows that foods rich in omega-3 fatty acids, fish, seafood, nuts, wild game, and seeds, are healthy. In particular, the consumption of fish has been associated with a reduction in killer diseases. Fish are rich in the omega-3 fatty acids known as EPA and DHA. These oils are highly desired by the cells for both structural and functional purposes. The brain readily incorporates them for use in brain cell growth and repair as well as nerve cell transmission. These oils are also needed by the heart and arteries. Here, they prevent clotting and fat build-up. The fish oils are a kind of natural antifreeze, that is they keep the blood in a fluid state, especially during the winter. They are also invaluable for cell walls, because they help keep these walls flexible, whereas excessive saturated fats may cause them to stiffen. It is a balance of both saturated fats and omega-3s which is ideal.

Only modest amounts of such oils are needed, for instance, one or two percent of total calories. Thus, it is unnecessary to eat fish daily. For most people twice a week is sufficient (even so, if all people did this, it would place enormous stress on the oceans, and they would quickly become depleted). The remainder of the meals may be traditional, that is red meat, lamb, poultry dishes, egg dishes, and vegetarian dishes. Certainly, fish can be eaten more often than this. However, there is a significant concern. First, the oceans are being depleted, and in some regions fish stocks are down some 90%. Thus, the entire ocean is at risk for extinction. What's more, ocean fish, especially large species, such as king salmon, tuna, halibut, swordfish, marlin, and bluefish, are heavily contaminated. Even the smaller fish are now contaminated.

The main contaminant is mercury. The levels of mercury in large ocean fish are so high that recent recommendations by the U.S. federal government call for restriction of intake. The newest guidelines are for large-sized salmon and/or tuna. They are to be eaten only once or twice per month. Otherwise, tissue and organ levels of mercury climb to toxic, in fact, life-threatening levels. At a recent medical meeting Michael Schechter, M.D., of New York reported an ominous finding: people who have restricted animal foods, replacing them with fish, have become mercury toxic.

By purposely replacing animal foods with fish, that is the increased intake of salmon, halibut, and tuna, these individuals were poisoning themselves, albeit unknowingly. In such patients Schechter, using chelation therapy, removed vast quantities of mercury, far more than was found in non-fish eaters. By attempting to do what was perceived as healthy these individuals were actually impairing their health. Thus, the consumption of large ocean fish should be restricted to one or two servings per month. There is a caveat. Apparently, canned tuna has less mercury than the fresh type. Thus, canned tuna may be eaten perhaps two or three servings per month. For pregnant women the recommendation is for even a lower intake, like once or twice per month. Also, there is a special high grade albacore tuna that is remote-source. Made from smaller tuna, this is delicious plus it is low in heavy metals (see Americanwildfoods.com).

Fish oils may be taken separately, that is as supplements. Companies screen their fish oil products for toxins, including heavy metals. The toxins and heavy metals can be cleansed through certain chemical processes. If taking fish oils, be sure to take only a type guaranteed free of heavy metals. Even so, these fish oils are heavily refined. This refining process requires the use of detergents, residues of which remains in the oils. In fact, the thirst for profits have driven fish oil makers to purge the oceans of its limited resources, all for the pursuit of a pharmaceutical agent.

Also, there is environmental damage related to the production of such oils. This leads to the depletion, if not collapse, of certain critical species such as salmon, bluefish, albacore tuna, and cod. However, now, there are alternatives. The oil derived from line-caught fish is one such option, particularly the oil extract of wild sockeye salmon. The sockeye salmon are smaller and, thus, are the lowest of all in mercury.

Another alternative is the oil derived from the Amazonian seed called sacha inchi. This seed is some 50% omega-3s by weight. This omega 3-rich oil is obtained by cold-pressing, ideally from the organically grown seed. Only sacha inchi oil can act as the ideal vegetarian replacement for fish oils by providing EPA and DHA precursors. Yet, it is unique when contrasted to fish oils, because it is completely wild and unrefined. This, along with wild sockeye salmon oil, is the highest quality and purest omega 3 source known.

Fish oils are usually preserved with genetically engineered ascorbic acid and vitamin E. Thus, they are extensively tainted. As well, detergents and solvents are used in processing. Thus, organically grown sacha inchi oil, this cold-pressed 'pure-omega,' is the cleanest and most environmentally friendly source of omega-3s available. It is the most ideal option for fish oil for those who refuse to consume animal foods.

What's more, ascorbic acid and vitamin E from genetically engineered sources have been proven toxic. Surely, no one takes supplements to become poisoned. In a study conducted by the *Lancet* by Poston and colleagues synthetic genetically modified vitamin C was found to increase the risks in pregnant mothers for stillbirths. John Hopkins found that people who took this corrupted vitamin E, which is from genetically engineered soy, gained no benefit, and, when the vitamin was taken in high doses, there was actually an increase in fatalities. In contrast, safe preservatives, actually healthy ones, for omega-3s are rosemary oil, sage oil, oregano oil, and natural vitamin C.

The only truly whole and low toxicity fish oil is the type derived from wild sockeye salmon. This is a highly nutritionally rich oil. This is the wild remote-source sockeye salmon from northern Alaska. Testing proves that it is exceptionally low in mercury, far lower than any other fatty fish. In fact, levels of toxins in such oil are so low that no refinement is necessary.

Pituitary types require significant amounts of omega-3s. This is because the omega-3s are of critical importance for brain function, including pituitary function. Essentially, these oils directly feed the pituitary, helping boost internal hormone function. For ideal results sacha inchi oil should be combined with the intake of remote-source fish oil such as wild Alaskan sockeye salmon oil. Both these oils greatly nourish the endocrine glands, particularly the pituitary and adrenal glands.

The majority of pituitary types are of northern European descent. This means that fatty fish, such as salmon, trout, herring, and sardines, are part of their native diet. The bodies of such people are geared for utilizing the fats from such fish. However, now the fish is contaminated, so it cannot be consumed in huge amounts. So, the alternative is to consume omega-3-rich oils free of such contaminants.

It must be reiterated that, today, with the exception of Alaskan sockeye salmon oil, and, perhaps, cold-pressed cod liver oil, which are low in heavy metals and which are unrefined, fish oils are not a natural product. Rather, they are pharmaceutical. Thus, they are highly refined. Some of the best sources of fish oils are also the ones that are severely contaminated. These include salmon, sardines, halibut, bluefish, albacore tuna, herring, trout and anchovies. The latest regulations are to reduce the consumption of large ocean fish, such as King Salmon, tuna, and halibut, to one or a maximum of two servings a month. This is because while the fatty fish oils are gland-nourishing, heavy metals readily poison the glands. Thus, in the event of heavy metal poisoning significant pituitary, adrenal, and thyroid disorders result.

Certain natural substances chelate, that is bind, heavy metals. One of the most effective of these is red sour grape. This is available commercially as red sour grape bulk powder or capsules. This is a burnt red/orange-appearing powder that is highly sour to taste. To purge heavy metals take two teaspoons of the flavonoid-rich sour grape concentrate twice daily or four capsules twice daily. The sour acids are highly binding against heavy metals. Also, natural-source vitamin C helps purge heavy metals. Another way to remove heavy metals is through purging the liver. This is through the intake of wild triple greens extracts as well as liver cell-boosting spice flushing agents such as the multiple spice oil complex in a base of extra virgin olive oil. This multiple spice oil complex contains oils of fennel, coriander, cumin plus heavy oils and wild greens. In addition, wild raw berries drops also help bind and purge toxic compounds. These extracts/formulas are sufficient to achieve liver cleansing.

Essential fatty acids: metabolic giants

The essential fatty acids are so named, because they are essential for life. All cell functions are dependent upon them. What's more, without them cells and, ultimately, organs degenerate. They are needed for daily existence. Severe deficiency may even result in death, especially in developing infants. Chemically, these essential substances are known as linoleic and linolenic acids. These fatty acids differ by the degree of one carbon atom. Linolenic is the more rare type. It is found primarily in nuts, wild fruit, wild game, and seeds. Both these fatty acids are found mainly in vegetable foods, although organ meats may contain small amounts. Wild game is also an excellent source. This is due to the diet of wild animals, which is high in nuts, seeds, and weeds plus certain fruit, especially wild berries, which are high in these fatty acids.

The essential fatty acids are one of the most potent stimulants of metabolism. Theses substances fit directly into the enzyme systems. Here, they activate the metabolism of all cells. In this regard they stimulate fat burning as well as cell development. They are also needed for the integrity of the skin, hair, nails, and joints.

Essential fatty acids are critical for hormone production. All glands are dependent upon them. However, they are particularly needed by the pituitary and adrenal glands. Regarding the latter because of their high rate of metabolism they quickly burn them up. Here, omega-3s, such as those found in organically grown sacha inchi oil, wild steam-extracted sockeye salmon oil, and berry seed essential fatty acids, are ideal. In particular, sacha inchi oil is thoroughly metabolized. Muscular types also require them, but it is the pituitary and thyroid types which are in the greatest need. Thus, for all types regular supplementation is mandatory. Here is an ideal supplemental program for the correction of essential fatty acid deficiency:

- crude pumpkinseed oil, Austrian source, fortified with fennel and rosemary oils: two to three tablespoons daily (also, eat the crude dark-skinned pumpkinseeds, salted as well as sprouted salted sunflower seeds. Note: see AmericanWildFoods.com)

- organically grown sacha inchi seed oil: one to three teaspoonsful daily

- wild Alaskan sockeye salmon oil: 2 or 3 capsules daily or one teaspoon daily.

- berry seed essential oils: 40 drops twice daily

Note: the combination of different types of oil sources is ideal, especially for the correction of severe or long-standing deficiencies. A more simple method may be taken such as merely taking only one of the aforementioned. Of these, the sacha inchi oil and wild sockeye salmon oil are ideal. Yet, again, for optimal results follow the complete program.

Fatty nutrients: key to endocrine health

The glands love fats. In fact, fatty foods provide much nourishment to the hormone systems. The fatty substances are the most nourishing of all nutrients to the endocrine system. Here, these materials act as major fuel sources. Also, fats, particularly the essential fatty acids and cholesterol, act for structural support in all cells. The combined intake of cholesterol-rich and essential fatty acid-rich foods, along with high-grade essential fatty acid supplements, effectively regulates the entire body.

The glands vigorously utilize fatty nutrients, particularly the fat soluble vitamins. There are two kinds of such vitamins: those which mix readily in water and those which mix only in fat. The former are known as water soluble vitamins, while the latter are known as fat soluble vitamins. It is the fat soluble vitamins which are the key to a strong hormone system. There is a third category: the pseudo-fat soluble vitamins. These vitamins are ultra-critical for proper glandular function. Found in fatty foods they are mainly soluble in water. Riboflavin is an example of such a vitamin. It is found primarily in the fatty portions of milk, cheese, and butter as well as in meats and fatty fish. While more rare in vegetables and fruit avocado, high in fat, contains a fair amount. Regarding vegetables wild greens are the exceptions, because these are an excellent source. An ideal supplemental source of riboflavin is a wild triple-greens flushing agent along with a special wild greens drink known as Super-5-Greens.

The germs of grains are also rich in fat-loving vitamins. Pantothenic acid is another water soluble vitamin found mainly in fatty foods. Top sources of this vitamin include the fatty germ of grain, whole milk products, egg yolks, fatty fish, organ meats, and fresh red meat. Thus, both riboflavin and pantothenic acid are a kind of fat soluble substance, that is they are generally only found in large amounts in fatty or protein-rich foods. The best sources of pantothenic acid are royal jelly, bee pollen, torula yeast, and rice bran.

The fat soluble vitamins were discovered in the 1920s, when researchers demonstrated substances in the fatty parts of food, which are necessary for cellular growth. They found that when animals were placed on a synthetic diet lacking this factor they degenerated. If this missing factor was added back to the diet, the animals thrived. Only four such factors are known: vitamins A, D, E, and K. However, certainly, within the fatty portions of foods there are numerous other growth factors, which have yet to be discovered. This is why nutritional supplements containing only the known factors fail to heal tissue as well as crude food fractions or the whole foods themselves. Remember, Dr. Westin Price cured a non-healing fracture with butter concentrate.

The pseudo-fat soluble vitamins include riboflavin and pantothenic acid. Incredibly, butter is a top source of this nutrient. Riboflavin would be a good addition to any vital extract. It, too, is required for cellular growth. So is pantothenic acid, which must also be used regularly for the proper growth and development of cells. As mentioned previously riboflavin is found naturally in wild greens extracts as well as torula yeast. Mountain grown or remote-source bee pollen is another key source. Even certain types of honey are also rich sources. For natural-source pantothenic acid rely upon triple strength royal jelly, torula yeast, and bee pollen.

Vitamin E: the hormone preservative

This vitamin is well known as an antioxidant. In the 1960s the Drs. Shute, Canadian M.D.s, popularized its value for heart disease. They may not have realized it, but the benefits discerned were probably largely due to its antioxidant actions. An antioxidant is a substance which, as the name implies, blocks oxidation. The oxidative process damages cells and accelerates aging. It can be compared to the rusting of a nail. When exposed to the elements, it oxidizes. Eventually, it becomes brittle and crumbles. Without protection, the same process occurs in the human body, again, through the actions of oxygen. The body, too, becomes tarnished through oxidation. Vitamin E blocks this. Through the regular intake of vitamin E the heart, being subject to a great amount of oxidation, is, therefore, preserved.

Vitamin E has a number of other actions, particularly related to hormones. It apparently acts as a preservative of hormones, extending their life span. This is why vitamin E-rich foods are so pervasive on this diet. Foods, such as nuts, seeds, sweet potatoes, seed oils, nut/seed butters, and organ meats, are major components of the metabolic diet. This is because wherever in food there is vitamin E there are also hormones. Thus, vitamin E-rich foods are among the most nourishing of all foods for hormone health.

Top food sources of this vitamin include sunflower seeds, pumpkin seeds, almonds, filberts, pecans, organic soybeans, salmon, sweet potatoes, crab, and lobster. The best supplemental source is sunflower seed vitamin E as capsules or oil (as drops under the tongue). Ideally, this should be in a base of wild red palm oil and crude pumpkinseed oil, both of which are top sources of this vitamin.

The importance of protein

Protein is critical to the human body. Many people are concerned about consuming excessive amounts of this substance, as if this could cause disease. This fear of protein has largely been perpetrated by the medical profession, which warns of possible organ damage from over-consumption. Yet, no proof is put forward of such an effect: just warnings and fear tactics. Thus, often, people view protein as a poison. How far removed human beings have become from the truth. The universal source, almighty God, made the protein molecule. Protein is required by every cell in the body. It is never poisonous. There can be imbalances created by too much protein, but this is usually mild. A far more serious issue is protein deficiency, which can lead to cell death as well as fatality.

All cells are made primarily of protein. In ancient times people ate mostly protein. Thus, how could it poison us? There is no need to fear it. What's more, whether a small amount, like a tiny steak, or a large amount, like a porterhouse, is eaten what difference would it make? It is all merely natural molecules, which the body utilizes. In contrast, a person drinks an artificially sweetened soft drink or perhaps eats chemically-infested ice cream or candy, without even considering the consequences. Such a person also eats pasta, rolls, and pastries routinely. Yet, this destroys the intestines as well as the rest of the organs. Natural food is constructive, that is it is utilized by the body to build new cells and to repair tissue. Synthetic substances destroy tissue and can never be used for rebuilding. Synthetic food always causes cellular damage. Also, protein from plants, especially grains, is surely no better than animal protein. In fact, there are far more toxins in plant proteins, that is the proteins of beans and grains, than in animal proteins. A person should be far more concerned about consuming, for instance, lecithin-rich kidney or mung beans or gluten-rich wheat or rye than organic beef or poultry.

There is no need to fear animal protein. If its role is understood, this helps eliminate fear. Here, it is first necessary to understand the chemical structure of such a substance. Proteins are a large number of related compounds, all of which are made from atoms of carbon plus nitrogen as well as sulfur. When proteins are digested, chains of these atoms are the main breakdown products.

These are the same atoms found in the air humans breathe. How could this be harmful? In fact, there is a greater degree of harm caused by a lack of protein than its excess. In all the years of practicing medicine I have never seen a single case of disease caused by excess protein. However, I have seen thousands of cases of disease, where excess sugar and starch cause organ damage, even death. I have also seen thousands of cases of disease due to protein deficiency. Truly, compared to other categories of food, people today eat a minimal amount of protein. What's more, compared to humankind's ancient ancestors the protein intake of modern man is minimal. Even today in primitive regions there are people who eat vast amounts of protein at which most Westerners would be aghast.

When an African slaughters an elephant, what does he do? He eats constantly vast quantities of meat. When an Inuit or northern Siberian slaughters a caribou, reindeer, or whale, what does he do? He eats his fill constantly, consuming all parts of the animal. Do any such people get sick? Do they get cancer? Do they die of kidney failure? Absolutely not. They are free of disease, rather, they are vital and powerful, that is until they start eating Westernized processed foods. In fact, it is the sugar and starch eaters who are dying of cancer and kidney disease. Americans live in fear. The thought of eating a large portion of protein frightens many. Today, if a person eats a large steak, often, there are bizarre thoughts. There could be fear of "illness." There could be guilt. There could even be shame. Americans are victims of propaganda. Such feelings are baseless.

Regardless of the condition protein cannot be arbitrarily removed from the diet without causing damage. Purposely restricting it is dangerous. In virtually all cases this will result in tissue damage and, ultimately, disease. In some people, especially thyroid types, such an approach will also result in a more dire consequence, which is an untimely death.

True, there are many dangerous high protein or animal foods. Examples include nitrated meats, sausages, and greasy chemically treated cold cuts. Commercial poultry is also dangerous. These cause significant damage. People are well aware of reports that meat eaters die younger and get more cancer than vegetarians. Yet, this is largely due to the type of meat that is consumed. People in the Western world read the reports of violent illnesses resulting from germ-contaminated meat. They read about the noxious substances given or fed to cattle, including hormones, pesticides, antibiotics, and other drugs. They eliminate meat, because they feel ill and are also afraid. Thus, it is largely justifiable that they would remove commercial meats from the diet. Yet, the key is the word *commercial*. Thus, rather than meat itself it is the way it is raised and processed that makes it toxic.

With the exception of pork, meat or milk products from organic sources have no major connection to disease. Thus, meat and other animal foods in their natural state are non-toxic. However, still, there is the desire to get well at any cost. The fear of disease and death causes people to take radical steps, and meat is the first victim of such thinking. However, in certain body types it is difficult if not impossible to follow a meat-free diet. Thus, with the endocrine type system a more liberal approach must be taken for food selection.

People may need to adopt a vegetarian diet in the treatment of certain diseases, notably cancer. In fact, in some situations such a diet could prove curative: colon cancer for instance. However, this should never be a permanent approach. It should be a short phase diet, like a vegetable and fruit cleanse, lasting, at most, a year or two or somewhat longer. Following such a diet for a more prolonged period can lead to cell death and organ damage. So, once the tissues are detoxified a more moderate diet must be followed. This is because extreme vegan and/or vegetarian diets, in fact, instigate certain cancers, especially lymphoma and leukemia. Such diets can also lead to heart attacks. A cure cannot be true if it also causes disease. Such diets also may result in liver disease, particularly cirrhosis, and this is particularly true in those who fail to properly manage their protein intake. Thus, such a strict diet, such as an extreme vegan diet, which is devoid of critical factors, including the essential amino acids, fat soluble vitamins, carnitine and vitamin B_{12}, must only be adhered to for a short period.

Proteins consist of compounds called amino acids. The word amino signifies the nitrogen content. It is the nitrogen which makes amino acids distinct from similar molecules such as vitamins. In contrast, vitamins consist mainly of carbon and may also contain sulfur and/or oxygen. Only the amino acids are nitrogen-based. There are eighteen common amino acids, which are listed as follows:

alanine	arginine
aspartic acid	cystine
glutamic acid	glycine
histidine	hydroxyglutamic acid
leucine	lysine
ornithine	oxyproline
phenlyalanine	proline
serine	tryptophan
tyrosine	valine

Protein is highly complex, far more complicated than mere vitamins and minerals. This consists of many building blocks. Protein is a higher compound, as it consists not only of amino acids but also 'built-in' vitamins and minerals. It is synthesized by animals from vegetation, that is cellulose. In this state it becomes a complete food. This is why of all foods the only kind that a person could subsist on wholly is animal protein. In other words, if a person only had one food and could only eat such a food, for instance, wheat and nothing else, fruit and nothing else, corn and nothing else: in all cases such a person would degenerate. However, if, in contrast, whole milk were the only food or pure organic beef, the individual could readily survive, even thrive, continuously (with cooked meat the problem of scurvy would ultimately arise, however). The point is that complete sources of amino acids are needed to maintain life.

If such sources are stripped from the diet, how can the individual thrive? It is difficult. The diet would need to be carefully constructed. The few vegetables which contain relatively complete proteins, such as almonds, soybeans, chick peas, hemp meal, and lentils, must form a significant part of the diet. High protein alternative 'grains,' particularly amaranth, quinoa, and teff, should be regularly consumed. It may not be possible. However, a deliberate effort must be made. In contrast, with animal foods it is far easier. All a person must do is include a few portions each week of healthy meats, eggs, or milk products and protein deficiency will never occur.

All proteins are different. They may be divided into strength-building proteins, intermediate proteins, and weak proteins. The strength-building types are capable of sustaining life. They are capable of causing the complete growth of cells. They are able to support the health of the organism, without defects. The intermediate types can largely do this, but they fail to support complete growth, especially in the developing young. If the weak or indigestible types are the only source of protein, defects will occur.

Strength-building proteins

Proteins which build strength are relatively few. These are the proteins of animal source, which contain all eight essential amino acids. The following are the most important protein sources to consume for the purpose of building tissue and maintaining overall health:

- milk (casein; lactalbumin, giving eight essential amino acids)
- meat (eight essential amino acids plus carnitine)
- egg (eight essential amino acids and sulfur-rich amino acids)
- fish (eight essential amino acids)
- poultry (eight essential amino acids plus carnitine)
- seafood (eight essential amino acids plus tissue salts)
- royal jelly (eight essential amino acids)

Intermediate proteins

- lentils
- wild rice
- brown rice
- beans (some)
- chlorella
- spirulina
- peanuts and peanut butter

- almonds
- filberts
- Brazil nuts
- pecans
- pine nuts
- amaranth
- quinoa
- tahini and sesame seeds
- garbanzo beans
- teff
- hemp meal
- brewers yeast and torula yeast

Low-level (weakening) proteins

- wheat (gluten)
- corn (zein)
- oats
- rye
- barley
- beans (some)

The proteins of the weak category can never provide the body's needs. Of these, the protein of oats is perhaps most considerable. Yet, if the weak proteins are ingested as the exclusive source, organ function may be devastated. Such proteins fail to fully nourish the tissues. Their only value is to prevent starvation. In fact, they should never be regarded as the exclusive protein source. Truly, if an individual attempts to survive on such foods, cellular starvation will result. The weak proteins actually deplete the protein stores, never replenishing them. What's more, certain of these, notably wheat and rye, destroy key nutrients needed for protein digestion, particularly zinc and phosphorus. They do so, because gluten-containing grains are high in compounds known as phytates. These compounds selectively bind zinc and phosphorus, preventing their absorption.

Gluten intolerance and zinc deficiency

Severe zinc deficiency is a common result from the overeating of grains, particularly wheat. This may be manifested by an obvious finding, which is multiple white spots or bands on the nails. Zinc is critical for protein digestion as well as for the building of protein.

People of the thyroid type have difficulty with digestion. So, the sticky gluten of grains presents an enormous challenge. It actually fails to digest, which invites an inflammatory response in the gut. This leads an immune reaction against the gut lining. The toxicity can be so great that the gut wall is virtually permanently damaged. Here, the absorptive surface of the gut is essentially demolished. This is known as gluten intolerance. Thus, with such wholesale destruction large minerals, such as zinc, fail to absorb. There is also malabsorption of vitamin A, which is needed for the absorption of this mineral. This explains the development of white spots on the fingernails.

The loss of zinc is devastating. The activity of dozens of enzymes are dependent upon this mineral. By destroying zinc and depleting the tissue stores of critical amino acids wheat protein causes cell damage. What's more, it can never build cells. Natural sources of zinc include crude wild oregano, organic red meat, wild game, bison, poultry, liver, kidney, pumpkin seeds, seafood, and eggs.

228 The Body Shape Diet

Rat experiments proved the danger. In the 1940s through 1960s these experiments proved that wheat protein is destructive to the tissues. Rats fed exclusively on wheat degenerated, failing to gain normal body weight. Visibly, they looked sick. Compared to healthy controls, who were fed strength-building proteins, such as the proteins of milk, their coat of hair was matted and sickly; they had a disheveled appearance. Their bones and joints were malformed, and they were scrawny. Their physiology, that is their organ function, was impaired. This means that the function of their digestive system was completely disrupted. Upon adding superior protein sources to their diet, such as whole milk or egg protein, these animals recovered. Then, are people to fear animal protein?

There is no doubt that grains are a poor source of nutrients. In particular, grains actually cause disease. This is particularly true of white flour. This was why the U.S. government forced Wonder Bread to destroy all billboards for false advertising, that is such bread not only fails to "Build Strong Bodies in Eight Ways," in fact, it destroys them. As a protein source bread, pasta, or similar wheat products offer no nutritional value. Nutritionally, they should be regarded as merely an accent to food. So, people should never rely upon them to supply the body's protein needs. Rather, they should be consumed mainly as a fuel and fiber source. However, crude whole grains do provide a significant amount of B vitamins. Yet, these B vitamins can be procured from non-grain foods such as brown rice, rice bran, wild greens, wild oregano crude herb, potato, vegetables, and meat.

Protein or starch: which is the enemy?

Again, people fear protein. This is ludicrous. In contrast, they never fear bread, pasta, wine, sweets, or ice cream. Yet, there is much to fear in such 'foods.' Protein is a natural substance, in fact, a very sophisticated one. Humans are incapable of making it, that is in the perfection found in nature. It is impossible to create complex proteins from scratch. No scientist has ever done so. How the body makes these proteins is a mystery. There are thousands of proteins in the body. Many of them are crucial for human survival. Protein is crucial for all cells.

With the exception of allergic reactions there is no evidence that the consumption of natural rich protein, such as the protein in red meat, eggs, or milk, causes any damage. Rather, evidence exists that poor quality protein, such as the form found in wheat, is destructive. Nor is there any evidence that animal protein shortens life span. In other words, protein molecules themselves are harmless. However, regarding the deficiency of this substance the evidence for dire effects is vast. Actually, millions of children die globally every year from protein deficiency. In contrast, none die from protein excess. Yet, for all such children starch is consumed in the excess, particularly by those who die prematurely.

The body requires protein. The cells completely require it. What's more, they require complete protein, that is the protein of fresh whole milk, eggs, red meat, poultry, and fish. This is what satisfies the cells the most. This is why human beings crave such proteins. The protein of grains, nuts, and seeds is acceptable, but it is far from preferred. In some cases it is completely rejected, for instance, in celiac disease. As mentioned previously in this condition the consumption of even a small amount of vegetable protein, usually as wheat, leads to wholesale cellular destruction. Incredibly, a single bite of bread, a roll, or pasta can cause the death of tens of millions or rather billions of cells. This is through the destruction of the gut wall. In contrast, with animal protein—even milk—no such destructive effects upon the gut wall are known. Again, the most destructive of all proteins to the intestinal system are the proteins of grains.

Here is the critical issue. Without protein, it is impossible to make hormones. This is because the breakdown products of protein, the amino acids, are required for hormone synthesis. Insulin, glucagon, thyroid hormone, parathyroid hormone, and adrenalin are all made from protein, that is amino acids. Pituitary hormones are also protein-based.

These hormones are highly complicated substances. They have a highly sophisticated three dimensional shape. It is impossible to make them, that is unless sufficient amino acids are supplied. This demonstrates the need for the regular intake of protein for all endocrine types. If there is a protein deficiency, there will also be a deficiency in hormone production. As a result of protein deficiency or the ingestion of malformed proteins all the organ systems are placed at risk.

Protein deficiency causes starvation. Recall the movies or documentaries of starving Africans? This is due to protein deficiency. Even in the Western world a kind of protein starvation is occurring. This is largely the result of trendy diets, which restrict protein intake. It is also the result of the excess consumption of sugar, which destroys protein. Plus, in diets rich in starchy foods its quality may be low, and this may lead to the deficiency. Protein is essential for life. Sugar and starch are non-essential.

The classical symptoms of protein starvation bear mentioning. These symptoms include swelling of the abdomen, the gaining of water weight, swelling of the feet, legs and/or ankles, hair loss, failure to grow or thrive, and loss of vitality.

The body type—the endocrine type—largely determines protein intake. For the thyroid type a high protein diet is indicated. Here, amino acids are needed for the synthesis of thyroid hormones. For the adrenal type the diet should be relatively high in protein and should also contain foods rich in cholesterol, like whole organic eggs, raw or whole organic milk products, particularly yogurt and cheese, seafood, fatty fish, and royal jelly. Here, a modest amount of complex carbohydrates can be consumed. For the pituitary type the diet should contain lesser amounts of protein—the metabolism is too slow—and plenty of vegetation, even fruit. Starch should be limited to the easy-to-digest varieties such as wild rice, potato with the skin on, amaranth, quinoa, and teff. The essential fatty acids found in nuts and seeds help balance pituitary hormone synthesis. Pituitary types also benefit from the brans of grains, including rice bran *but not the starch*. They need the density of B vitamins in the bran to activate the gland. In the thyroid-adrenal type the diet should be high in protein and fat plus some whole grains/starch. In the adrenal-thyroid type the protein is also important but, as well, a modest amount of starch can be consumed, and fat should be consumed liberally.

There is a danger in excessive restriction of protein. Even so, it is not that massive amounts must be consumed. It is just that a certain amount is needed for the proper function of the endocrine system—and some types need more protein than others. Much of the protein needs can be achieved through the daily intake of concentrated (3x) royal jelly.

Protein is crucial for the growth and development of all cells. It is required for the synthesis of thousands of essential compounds: enzymes, hormones, neurotransmitter, muscle proteins, genetic material, and more. For adrenal and pituitary types the raw amino acids and hormones found in royal jelly and high quality bee pollen, also found in smaller amounts in crude raw honey, are a boon. For optimal results use an undiluted 3x royal jelly, fortified with wild rosemary and sage. Do not accept cheap imitations.

Thus, in reasonable quantities it is useful to the body, never toxic. This is the normal physiology. The main types which benefit from a high protein diet are the thyroid type, the thyroid-adrenal type, and the muscular-thyroid type. The latter should have healthy servings of protein for each meal, along with vegetables. For energy it is better for this type to rely upon plenty of fruit instead of bread, pastries, and pasta.

So, in summary the various types should have the following diet (in general):

- thyroid type: mostly protein, dark green leafy vegetables, low-carbohydrate vegetables, plus eggs, whole milk products, nuts, and seeds; some fruit is allowed. Avoid cruciferous vegetables such as broccoli, cauliflower, cabbage, and Brussels sprouts (OK if cooked)

- adrenal type: protein plus fats and high cholesterol foods, including whole milk products and eggs, along with fresh fruit, whole grains, potatoes with the skin on, wild rice, whole grain rice products, nuts, seeds, and lesser amounts of vegetables (all starches should be salted) plus royal jelly

- pituitary type: remote-source fatty fish, seafood, white fish, small portions of animal protein, liver, organic turkey, nuts, seeds, vegetables, the brans of grains, whole organic eggs, wild rice, whole milk goat yogurt, and feta cheese

- muscular type: high protein (animal food), whole organic eggs, organic whole milk products, low starch vegetables, and fruit plus raw honey (for energy)

These are general rules—a basic guide. The section on each endocrine type provides greater detail on the exact nature of the diet plus supplementation. The recipes in the recipe section also act as a guide. Follow this, and the result will be superior health. That is the endocrine body shape guarantee.

Is meat good to eat every day?

In ancient times people were mainly meat eaters. There were little other sources for foods. Grains had yet to be developed. Even so, obviously, these ancients could never have eaten meat every day. Some days they had no food. Regardless, an all meat diet is highly restrictive. What's more, it is a good idea to fast from meat, for instance, for two or three days or even a week. During this fasting the ideal food to eat is fruit, another food of ancient man.

Fruit has a cleansing action on the organs, including the blood and intestines. If your plan calls for considerable amounts of meat, go without it for a day every week or two. Eat instead the food that is allowed, with nuts as a source of strength, if necessary. The fruit is highly cleansing and neutralizes any noxious effects of excessive meat. However, never attempt an all-fruit diet for prolonged periods. This is

234 The Body Shape Diet

particularly true for adrenal and pituitary types, as this could prove disastrous. Just eat nothing but fruit or fruit juices for a day or two: maximum. Then, continue the consumption of the appropriate amount of meat, eggs, whole milk products, nuts, and seeds to ensure adequate protein intake. Regardless, for any person who eats meat regularly such a one should be sure to neutralize any imbalances with plenty of wild berries or their extracts such as the wild raw eight berries drops.

Does meat cause cancer?

There is some evidence for a meat-cancer connection. However, this is true only of processed or commercial meats. Meat is only poisonous based upon the way it is raised. The exception is pork and chicken. Regardless of how these are raised there is a degree of danger. Of course, true free range chicken might be an exception. Even so, when cooking chicken, always add plenty of spices, because these destroy the toxins.

The flesh of animals which eat food other than grass is poisonous. This is particularly true of pork. For this meat there is a massive cancer connection. There is also a connection to diseases of the brain and spinal cord, notably ALS, multiple sclerosis, and Alzheimer's disease. Also, with commercially raised poultry there is a cancer connection, as published by the scholarly Virginia Livingston-Wheeler, M.D. She proved that commercial poultry contains cancer-causing viruses as well as carcinogenic bacteria. These viruses and bacteria were particularly concentrated in chicken livers. Yet, they were also found in the eggs. Thus, the cancer connection of commercial pork and poultry is real. In contrast, there is no known cancer connection with healthy meats, that is the meat of natural herbivores.

A number of studies have shown that the idea of healthy meat as poisonous has no basis. In other words, pure fresh red meat does not seem to cause any disease. Consider a study done by the *JAMA* (2005) and headed by Ann Chao, Ph.D., regarding diet and colon cancer. While processed meat definitely was associated, eating plain red meat did not increase the risks for this disease. Another study published in the *European Journal of Clinical Nutrition* made the same finding, which is that merely eating red meat did not cause colon cancer.

Again, regarding the ingestion of organic red meat in moderation there is no evidence of a cancer connection. However, processed meat, that is meat preserved with colorings and nitrates, clearly is connected. Also, truly organically fed poultry, as well as truly organic eggs, is far safer for human consumption than the commercially raised types. Regarding pork there is no safe type. Plus, spiritually, it is toxic.

Even so, in cancer little meat if any is needed. This is because meat provides putrefactive proteins, as well as blood cells, which may cause the cancer to grow. Most of this negative effect of meat can be neutralized by adding prodigious amounts of spices to the meats, which halt putrefaction. Here, a person can even add the spice oils to the food or marinade such as the oil of wild oregano, rosemary, sage, cumin, and cilantro (in an extra virgin olive oil base). This approach increases the safety of meat for cancer victims. Even so, many cancer patients thrive on a meat-free or meat-reduced diet. They even go into total remission or cure on such a diet, a fact which is indisputable. With active cancer the iron in meat seems to feed tumor growth.

However, a meat-free diet is not for everyone. Even certain cancer patients thrive when a reasonable amount of meat and/or fish is included. Again, the problem with meat in cancer is that meat juices can feed the tumor, acting as a growth factor. This may be due to the naturally occurring hormones in meat. In contrast, phytochemical-rich vegetation helps block tumor growth. Regardless, as a rule red meat should be avoided, that is until the cancer is cured. Spices are anti-cancer. They reduce or neutralize any cancer-stimulating effects. Plus, spices stimulate the immune system to fight the cancer. Also, when fixing meat dishes add plenty of garlic and onion, which are also anti-tumor.

The body needs amino acids. Thus, at a minimum organic beef, fish, or turkey broth may be needed by cancer victims. To exclude meat totally can be dangerous. With red meat it must be cooked lightly. Ideally, it should be medium-rare or even rare. Well done meat contains a greater amount of carcinogens than the blood-red. Regarding the broth this would be an ideal addition to the cancer-fighting diet. In curing cancer organic milk products are invaluable and are superior to meat. Organic yogurt, quark, cottage cheese, and kefir are all ideal. In active cancer it is necessary to avoid cheese, since fungi, which are contaminants of cheese, accelerate the growth of tumor cells. Also, the fungi suppress the immune system.

If consuming no meat, be sure to consume some other protein-rich food—for strength—for instance, bee pollen, royal jelly, and organic milk products. Also, cancer victims should consume large amounts of organically grown sacha inchi oil, combined with organic cottage cheese, quark, or yogurt. The organic sacha inchi oil can be poured over the milk products. This is the famous Yohanna Budwig plan, which is used successfully in Europe in the cure of cancer.

Also, realize that a vegetable-only diet starves the adrenal glands. This can lead to physiological collapse. Thus, for adrenal body types be sure to consume some sources of protein to neutralize excessively alkaline foods such as bee pollen, organic milk products, and royal jelly as well as an organic meat broth. The latter can be sipped on as a source of strength in cancer patients. Perhaps even superior is wild sockeye salmon oil, Alaskan-source, about a tablespoon daily.

Nutrients as hormones—the power of vitamins A and D

Vitamins have hormone-like properties. Two of the most powerful hormone-like vitamins are the fat soluble nutrients, vitamins A and D. These substances are found exclusively in fatty foods, mainly of animal origin. This is why animal foods, if from good, clean sources, help build physical strength. It will be noted that numerous animals crave fatty foods and particularly, when they capture prey, consume the fatty portions. These fatty portions are rich in various hormones and their precursors. They are also rich in the hormone-like nutrients, vitamins A and D.

Vitamin A: hormone precursor

Vitamin A is needed for the production of virtually all hormones. It is found in its pre-hormone form exclusively in animal foods. Thus, a complete lack of intake of animal-source foods rapidly leads to the deficiency. For hormone health this is disasterous, because this vitamin is involved in the synthesis of dozens of endocrine secretions.

The habits of polar and grizzly bear are revealing. After capturing an animal these bear eat mainly organ meats. For grizzlies when catching fish the head and entrails are its treat. Usually, the flesh or muscle is discarded. These animals are procuring the pre-hormone precursors found in these organs, which are not found in significant amounts in muscle. Thus, hormones give them strength. So, merely eating lean steak or chicken breast gives only a modest amount of pre-hormones. Yet, the skin of chicken and turkey—and the skin/organs of fatty fish, as well as the fatty fish drippings—are loaded in these precursors. So, only certain animal foods provide them. The animal foods which are rich in vitamin A and other pre-hormones include fatty fish, especially the skin and the tissue just under the skin, lobster, crab, clams, oysters, liver, sweetbreads, the skin of poultry, fatty duck, milk, cream, butter, and kidney. In the plant kingdom bee pollen, raw honey, kelp, maca root, nut/seed oils, and avocados contain such precursors. Yet, the plant forms are often different than those found in animals. There is, however, no vitamin A in such foods.

A natural and safe animal source of vitamin A is available. This is the wild Alaskan sockeye salmon oil. This is a powerful source of this critical nutrient. It is available as an oil in an eight-ounce bottle and also as fish gelatin capsules. The vitamin A in these supplements is entirely natural and, in fact, wild.

"Hormone" D

The term vitamin D is a misnomer. This substance is a lipid, the same general molecule as estrogen and adrenal steroids. In fact, vitamin D is a steroid hormone. This is because it is produced within the body and secreted into the blood, which is the definition of a hormone. In contrast, a vitamin is an essential substance, which is impossible to produce in the body, and which must therefore be procured through the diet. Yet, since it meets some of both definitions this substance is more correctly described as a vitamin-hormone.

Again, vitamin D can be made in the skin as a result of the action of sunlight. The raw material for making it is cholesterol. The sun strikes the skin, irradiating cholesterol molecules trapped within it. This converts these molecules to vitamin D, which is then transported into the blood and from here to all cells. Then, like a true hormone this substance enters the nucleus of the cell, where it exerts its action. The amount of time needed to form sufficient vitamin D varies with the color of the skin. For light colored people 15 minutes is sufficient to begin formation, while in darker skinned people this may vary from a half hour to several hours. Yet, it is possible to receive too much of a good thing. Particularly in light-skinned people staying in the sun for prolonged periods, especially if barely covered, is destructive to vitamin D production. This is because excessive ultraviolet light, in fact, destroys skin cells, the very cells which produce this hormone.

The main purpose of vitamin D is to control calcium metabolism and, particularly, the deposition of this mineral into bone. Bone health is completely dependent upon this hormone, because the absorption of calcium from the intestines is largely controlled by this substance. Sunlight stimulates the production of this crucial hormone, as long as the skin isn't burned.

Calcium itself is a crucial anti-cancer substance. It helps regulate cell growth. A high calcium intake is greatly protective against cancer. This may explain the observation that a high vitamin D intake prevents this disease. It may also explain why regular exposure to sunlight significantly reduces cancer risks. It may also be the reason that people who regularly eat milk products have a lower risk of colon cancer than those who fail to eat them.

How to increase hormone levels: the power of fasting

Great men in the past have left pearls of wisdom. It was the Prophet Muhammad who originated the first system of fasting. This system offers remarkable benefits for overall health. Studies have shown that fasting—through the Islaamic method—causes a significant rise in the levels of sex hormones in the body. The study, performed by S. Abbas and published in *Archives of Andrology,* determined that the Islaamic fast caused an increase in sperm count and also increased the blood levels of beneficial sex hormones. Levels of both pituitary and testicular hormones (testosterone) rose.

Some 1.4 billion people do this. Such a fast preserves the tissues, greatly increasing longevity. The almighty creator loves His creation. So, He offers much good to them. Though there is a sacrifice involved, mere abstinence, the gains are great. The increase in sperm counts, for instance, during the Islaamic fast indicates that it induces a kind of biological synthesis. Fasting, said the Prophet, is the best medicine.

Thus, fasting acts as a preservative, which allows the body to rebuild. This has been recently confirmed by Walford and his group, who found that caloric restriction is a potent cure for a variety of diseases. This includes the potential reversal of old age. Through regular fasting Walford has determined that life span can be significantly increased. It is an ideal way to systematically bolster hormone levels. This is because it leads to regeneration of the glands. Allen Cott, M.D., in his book *Fasting: The Ultimate Diet* quotes Russian physician Yuri Nikoloyiv, who cured the vast majority of his patients simply through fasting. The resting of the gut is a powerful regenerative. It is effective if done regularly, such as the yearly Islaamic fast.

Hormones which dramatically rise from fasting include levels of insulin, cortisone, aldosterone, testosterone, progesterone, estrogen (the healthy kinds), melatonin, and DHEA. Fasting increases the hormone reserve of all organs. Thus, it decreases the stress and strain on these organs, while improving their resistance to disease.

The human glands are readily depleted. This is particularly true for those enduring prolonged stress. Fasting is an efficient means to regenerate these glands, allowing much needed supplies to be replenished.

People of all body types benefit from this. Thus, it is beneficial to adopt a form of safe, systematic fasting such as the Islaamic fast. Humans in general have no discipline. This fast creates the routine of discipline for the benefit of the individual. There is no escaping it. There is no procrastination. Every year, there must be a fast.

The fast is simply no food or drink until sunset. Thus, this rests the entire digestive system. Any food or drink—even water—activates the digestive organs as well as the endocrine glands. Even the mechanical stimulation from food distresses the hormone system, as does, particularly, the various chemicals in food. Total abstinence is the only method for causing regeneration. This is why during the fasting period nothing must be consumed. The benefit of this once a year fast for approximately 30 days is a longer, healthier life. Voluntary fasts after this help maintain the benefits.

Vital iodine: thyroid and ovarian activator

The role of iodine in thyroid function is well known. However, what is less well understood is its role as a vitality factor: for the entire body. The emphasis has always been its role in thyroid function, where it is essential. However, this invaluable nutrient feeds a wide range of organs and tissues. White blood cells use it as an antiseptic for killing microbes. In the ovaries and testes it is used to stimulate cell synthesis as well as to protect these organs against germs. Iodine activates bone chemistry, aiding in the deposition of calcium. It is also an activator of the bone marrow, where it boosts the synthesis of white blood cells.

It may also act as an intracellular preservative, that is an anti-aging factor. Cultures where iodine intake is high, such as the people of Japan and Okinawa, have among the longest life spans in the world. In fact, the regular intake of iodine has more to do with the vital health of these people than perhaps any other factor. It may also play a role in their inherent productivity. The Japanese are among the most energetic of all peoples. Iodine activates thyroid hormone.

What's more, this hormone activates brain cells. Thus, it is easy to realize how iodine-rich foods are key for maintaining a powerful hormone status. This may explain the significant increase in longevity seen in various regions of Japan such as Okinawa. It also explains why the people of the region are traditionally slender.

This substance is found extensively in nature. It may be depleted in certain regions, that is in the soil and water. The iodine in nature is derived chiefly from weathered rocks from mountains. Mountain streams essentially deliver this where it is needed: the valleys and river-ways. The water filters into the soil or aquifers, bringing this element within human reach. The water from such rivers is evaporated, carrying the iodine with it. Then, it is redeposited into the earth and soil through the rain. Thus, the cycle is completed, so that humans can benefit from this critical element. This is because without iodine life is impossible.

Despite this natural iodine cycle certain regions are severely deficient in this substance. The Alpine region is one of the most deficient. This is despite the fact that the rocky soil and rocks in the Alps contain this mineral. However, Kahn notes that the reason the region is lacking is that the water rushes down these mountains so quickly that there is no chance for the mineral to be deposited. Instead, it ends up in the oceans or in lower elevations. Thus, people living in these mountains, who subsist mostly on local foods, and who drink this local water, are deficient. This is why goiter is incredibly common in these regions. The introduction of iodized salt dramatically reduced the incidence of goiter in the Alpine regions.

Thus, the rivers drive the iodine from the rocks and soil into the ocean. Over tens of millions of years the oceans have become a veritable iodine soup. Ocean plants, fish, and seafood concentrate this mineral and, thus, become a human's iodine supplements. The richest fish sources are cod and haddock. In contrast, herring is low. Cod liver oil, especially the unrefined variety, is exceptionally rich. However, now it is difficult if not impossible to find the unrefined type. An optional source for natural fish-based iodine is unrefined wild sockeye salmon oil.

When water is evaporated from the oceans, a certain amount of iodine, which is gas-like, is vaporized. This is returned to the earth via rain. Ultimately, through both the wearing of rock and iodine-rich rain the soil becomes enriched in this mineral. Plants take it up, the plants are eaten by animals, and the cycle continues. This is why certain flesh, particularly beef, is high in this nutrient. Of the various vegetables garlic has the highest content. In fact, garlic is some four times richer in this nutrient than onions. Other common foods which are relatively rich include bison, elk, venison, lamb, grass-fed beef, radishes, turnips, eggs, milk, and butter.

The human body contains a relatively small amount of this nutrient. It is poorly stored, so it must be constantly replenished. A fair amount of this nutrient circulates in the blood to fulfill the needs particularly of the thyroid and ovaries. It is also concentrated in the liver. During agitation or excitement the iodine content of the blood goes up; it is poured out by the glands. It also rises during the menstrual cycle. The ovaries need it for dealing with menstrual stress. Without this mineral menstrual actions are depressed. The period is sluggish, the flow is scanty or excessive, and there is weight gain, cramps, and breast tenderness. All this is reversed by adding sufficient iodine into the diet.

Again, most of the iodine found in the body is concentrated in the endocrine glands, although the muscles also contain a considerable amount. The ovaries are second only to the thyroid in iodine content, a fact which is rarely appreciated. Thus, disorders of the female sex glands may often be related to iodine deficiency.

The pituitary and adrenal glands also concentrate this nutrient. The thyroid contains the greatest amount and is the chief agent of iodine metabolism. Here, iodine is bound with an amino acid, tyrosine, to form thyroid hormone.

In nature there is an enormous effort to bring iodine within human reach. Rain moves it, as does evaporation. Of course, all the seas are iodine-rich, especially all regions of the Atlantic and Pacific Oceans. This demonstrates the critical importance of this substance, not just for the thyroid gland but for all organ systems. There is a deliberate effort to make iodine available, all for the sake of humanity as well as other creatures.

Light: an essential nutrient?

The endocrine glands are activated by light. In contrast, darkness causes them to become quiescent. Rather, a lack of sunlight, if prolonged, greatly depresses these glands. Therefore, light is essential for their function. It is equally important as a nutrient as any vitamin or nutrient.

The pituitary itself is highly light sensitive. Anatomically, it is positioned just below the light-receiving optic nerve. This region would appear to be the center of life. It is how the sensation of life enters the body. Thus, it is just as important in the balancing of metabolism as are nutrients and food. It was John Ott, one of the world's most premier researchers on the health benefits of light, who made it clear that without light, in particular, the full-spectrum light from the sun human life would be impossible. Said Ott, "Light entering the eyes influences the endocrine system, thereby influencing the production and release of hormones for the control of body chemistry..." Furthermore, he notes how light is a form of energy. This energy directly influences brain and gland function.

In Ott's early experiments it was determined that light therapy, that is the use of artificially produced full spectrum light, even aided certain diseases. Hyperactive children, as well as those with learning disabilities, responded remarkably well. The researchers also noted that regular exposure to natural daylight eased emotional problems as well as depression. The latter would indicate a direct action of the light on the endocrine glands. Yet, Ott's work ultimately became even more dramatic: he proved that the typical indoor light, both incandescent and fluorescent, in fact, causes disease. In his laboratory experiments he produced virtually every known major disease by altering animals' light sources and by routinely exposing them to indoor lighting. What's more, Ott's work was evaluated on humans, in this case cancer victims. By exposing the cancer patients to natural light and by reducing their exposure to synthetic light significant improvement was noted. Some patients went into remission.

Light is a major force in regulating hormonal actions. Even the sex glands appear to be regulated by it. Both male and female hormonal cycles normally are balanced through sunlight. Yet, as was proven by Germany's F. Hollwich so is adrenal function. Reasoning that the true effect of sunlight could be detected in blind people he actually studied people with cataracts. In evaluating some 250 people he found bizarre disturbances in physiology, all of which could be tied to adrenal dysfunction. Thus, the lack of natural light caused the adrenal glands to falter. Among the disturbances observed by Dr. Hollwich included blood sugar disorders, electrolyte imbalances, and inability to control fluid balance. The entire metabolism was disturbed. However, after the cataracts were removed much of these functions normalized.

For certain light activates the brain. As a result, the entire nervous system benefits. However, light is focused within the key hormonal regions. These key regions are the hypothalamus, pineal, and pituitary. All these organs respond to it. They require it for proper activation. For their hormones and messengers in these organs to be produced, they must be stimulated by light. Without sunlight or artificial forms of such light the output of these master glands dramatically declines. As a result, the entire body suffers. Thus, exposure to sunlight or artificially produced sunlight is essential in any endocrine recovery plan. So is the ingestion of wild raw berries or their extracts, as well as extracts of wild raw remote-source greens, which consist of elemental sunlight.

Lysine: hormone-nourishing amino acid

Lysine is of enormous importance for endocrine function. Thus, foods rich in this amino acid are of critical importance in regeneration. The importance of lysine was highlighted decades ago by the finding that if it is withdrawn from the diet, growth is stunted.

Lysine needs vary greatly, depending upon metabolism. A person with sluggish, as well as excessively rapid, metabolism requires additional supplies. There may be as much as ten-fold variations between individuals regarding the cellular needs. Lysine may be metabolized to a substance known as coenzyme A, which is critical to carbohydrate metabolism. Thus, diets rich in this amino acid help stimulate weight loss.

The metabolism of lysine is dependent upon other nutrients, notably niacin, riboflavin, and vitamin C. It is used primarily in the body to form connective tissue, particularly the collagen linings of the joints. However, there is another critical use. This is the production of carnitine. The synthesis of the latter is entirely dependent upon lysine. It is carnitine which is so essential to hormone metabolism. The fact is no major lipid-based hormone can be activated, let alone enter the cell, without it. Carnitine is a specialized molecule: it is a kind of cellular truck-driver, transporting its load, usually fatty acids, directly into the cells.

Top food sources of lysine include cottage cheese, whole milk, red meat, eggs, ricotta cheese, yogurt, turkey, duck, and whole oats. These are also the best sources of carnitine. Regarding the cereal sources of lysine oat bran is preferred, since it is far more dense in this amino acid than oatmeal. Wild game is the richest source. Except for soy and maca root there are no significant vegetable sources for this nutrient. A lack of lysine may explain another cause of human degeneration: herpes infection. Such infections are commonly represented by cold sores. Supplemental lysine has been found to prevent them. Researchers discovered that lysine blocks herpes virus growth, while another amino acid, arginine, stimulates it. Arginine is an antagonist to lysine. It is found largely in grains, beans, nuts, and legumes. Eating such foods can aggravate or even cause cold sores. In particular, peanuts, which are high in arginine and relatively low in lysine, provoke herpes attacks. For those who are vulnerable to herpetic and/or cold sore attacks it is advisable to avoid nuts and opt for animal sources of protein such as poultry, organic beef, lamb, organic whole milk, yogurt, and farm fresh or organic eggs. The aforementioned are top dietary sources of lysine. Wheat and corn are poor sources.

Phospholipids: nature's emulsifiers

Emulsifiers are of value to the human body. Everyone knows that fat and water don't mix. Yet, the body is mostly water: enter the power of emulsifiers. It is these agents which cause the fat and water to blend, much like the blending which exists in milk. The body has its own fatty milk. This is the lymph. It is the emulsifiers which are responsible for such a blending. In fact, fat is largely absorbed and transported through the lymphatics. This is critical, since hormones are also largely fat, and they, too, are transported in the milky lymph.

The lymph is the front line of defense of the body against toxicity and infection. For it to be effective it must be in this milky, creamy state, and this is accomplished through naturally occurring emulsifying agents. Lecithin, a phospholipid, is the main naturally occurring emulsifier. An emulsifier is a substance capable of breaking fat globules into tiny components to make them easier to absorb. Thus, these agents are used in the food industry for blending fats into water, for instance, in the making of pudding and ice cream. Yet, incredibly, cholesterol is equally if not more important in fat blending. The body uses it to even cause the absorption of fat, that is through the bile.

This proves the importance of including heavy fats, including animal fat, in the diet. Animal fat is the main source of lecithin. Another source is the cold-processed oils of nuts and seeds as well as soybeans (which are legumes). However, in vegetation there is no cholesterol and little lecithin. True, lecithin is found in nuts and seeds, as well as soy, but there is no cholesterol in vegetables or fruit. There are plant sterols, but as is demonstrated by plant-sterol based drugs these are difficult to absorb. In fact, they are cholesterol antagonists, meaning they block cholesterol absorption. Vegetable sources of emulsifying agents include fatty seed oils (cold-pressed) such as black seed oil, sesame oil, extra virgin olive oil, and avocado oil. Yet, even so it is the animal foods that contain actual hormones as well as a significant amount of pre-hormones. With the exception of kelp and bee pollen in vegetation such substances are rare.

Lecithin, as well as cholesterol, are "important participant(s) in fat digestion..." Egg yolks are the richest source of both these substances. Thus, they are the ideal source for naturally occurring emulsifiers. This is only true of partially cooked or raw egg yolks. Thorough cooking inactivates this function. Only organic egg yolks in a relatively fluid state must be consumed. Thus, when cooking eggs, they must be cooked soft boiled or 'over easy.'

The liver is the hub of all cell synthesis. It is also the center for fat digestion and absorption. It depends mainly upon two substances to achieve the latter. These substances are lecithin and cholesterol. Thus, these two substances are critical components of the diet, since fat is essential to the cells: all cells. For a long and vigorous life a person must eat prodigious quantities of it. Cholesterol is found in every cell in the body. It is a main component of cell walls. It is the key molecule for maintaining the health of nerve cells. Cholesterol is critical for human life.

When cholesterol levels decline precipitously, cellular death results. This is a testimony against forcibly lowering cholesterol levels. In fact, rather than fearing it there should be a fear of lacking it. This is the opposite of what people are taught. For ideal health this substance must be ingested in the form of healthy milk products, which are ideally eaten raw, yogurt, natural/organic eggs, organic meats, organic poultry, seafood, and fatty fish.

To strictly avoid cholesterol is to court disaster. This is because it results in cell exhaustion, endocrine collapse, cell death, and sudden demise. Thus, for optimal health it is necessary to eat rich sources of cholesterol. By adding cholesterol- and lecithin-rich foods regularly into the diet a major difference will be noticed immediately. Plus, such foods are tasty and rich, that is they are enjoyable. God made it that way; why not take advantage of it? The best sources of cholesterol are eggs, kidney, liver, heart, shrimp, lamb, crab, beef, lobster, chicken, turkey, halibut, tuna, salmon, cream, whole milk, and cheese, basically in descending order. These foods are also the best sources of lecithin. Regarding lecithin nuts, seeds, whole soybeans, and avocados are excellent sources, but, again, such foods are devoid of cholesterol. Also, it is difficult to get quality soy, since virtually all commercial soy is genetically engineered. Such soy is unfit for human consumption. Then, so is the lecithin derived from such soy. A raw wild nut milk made from hickory nuts, which is rich in lecithin, is also available (see exclusively Americanwildfoods.com).

The lecithin which is found in vegetation is less bioactive than the animal type. Remember, in water fats and oils never mix. From an endocrine point of view eating merely vegetables and fruit is an inadequate diet. In such a diet there is no means for the naturally occurring fats to be absorbed. So, too, will the absorption of fat soluble vitamins fail. Thus, routinely mainly vegetable eaters are grossly deficient in vitamins A and D. To remain in ideal health they must supplement the diet with those nutrients.

For optimal health, particularly related to the hormone system, it is critical to eat a variety of fatty foods. Examples of such foods are found in the recipe section. These foods can be eaten as a regular part of the diet, especially those which naturally contain the emulsifying agents, cholesterol and lecithin.

Then, the body is mainly water. The liver cannot properly function in an exclusively watery environment. It is only fatty foods which make the liver work and which, in fact, exercise it. Fat forces the liver to work by causing it to make bile. By restricting fat the liver becomes stagnant, which can lead to internal degeneration. In fact, when the bile levels become exceedingly low, the remaining bile becomes sticky, clinging to the inside of the liver and gallbladder. This gluey bile causes inflammation and, ultimately, infection. Calcium may be deposited, leading to gallbladder attacks, gallstones, and liver disease. Such a condition is common, particularly in the thyroid and thyroid-adrenal types, since such individuals suffer from sluggish liver metabolism.

The importance of this process, that is this emulsification of fat, is beyond comprehension. It is one of the most critical processes in the body. This human body requires fat, and the organs must be supported to digest it. This support is through the intake of cholesterol-rich and lecithin-rich foods. It is also through the consumption of reasonable amounts of fat. Skimping on the fat greatly reduces fat absorption, which leads to a vast array of deficiencies. There are dozens of key fats and fatty acids required by the body. These are known as fat soluble nutrients. The fat soluble nutrients include vitamins A, D, E, and K, coenzyme Q-10, choline, inositol, essential fatty acids, sterols, beta carotene, lycopene, flavonoids, phenols, and lecithin as well as cholesterol itself. If fat is removed or restricted from the diet, it is difficult if not impossible for such nutrients to be absorbed.

For optimal health fat is absolutely critical. It is far from evil. No one should arbitrarily avoid it. In fact, to gain ideal health there should be an effort to regularly include it in the diet. What's more, to have a powerful hormone system, especially powerful adrenal glands and sex glands, its intake is crucial. For many adrenal types a rich intake of fat is critical, especially in the form of cholesterol and its precursors.

However, the greatest beneficiaries of a high fat diet are people with thyroid and also adrenal syndromes. Here, the regular intake of fat helps rest the glands by decreasing the metabolic rate. Also, the natural fat in food contains hormones and their precursors as well as the much needed fat soluble vitamins. Furthermore, fat stimulates the flow of bile, which is crucial for the optimal function of the glandular system. This is why a low fat diet may lead to degeneration of the endocrine glands, particularly the thyroid, adrenals, testes, and ovaries.

Chapter Seven

The Brain: A Metabolic Organ?

The brain controls metabolism. It is the center of all metabolism, because it houses three key endocrine organs, which are the hypothalmus, pineal gland, and pituitary gland. A person can improve the metabolism through brain power. In other words it is possible to *think* power into the endocrine glands. This can be done through relaxation techniques as well as positive thinking. So, if a person has a specific weakness, then, mental therapy can be successfully used. Such a one must talk to his/her glands and tell them to be healthy. They can be commanded to act powerfully. This is because, ultimately, it is the brain which controls hormone secretion.

It is important to think positively. All functions in these glands are tied to the nervous system. Even the brain is under endocrine control. Thus, it is no surprise that diseases/disorders of the glands are often confused with mental disease. In other words, anxiety, panic attacks, depression, manic-depressive syndrome, and even schizophrenia may all be primary endocrine disorders.

Mental disease is diagnosed as being exclusively related to the brain. This is an error. Incredibly, the brain has little if anything to do with it. In fact, the majority of mental diseases are due to factors exclusive to the brain. The brain itself may be involved, but usually it is not the primary factor. For instance, the brain is readily infected. Such an infection may cause depression and anxiety. It may also cause memory loss. There can also be nutritional deficiencies. There may also be hormonal deficiencies or imbalances, which directly impact this organ. This is why drug therapy, as well as psychotherapy, usually fail to cure mental diseases. The drugs have no positive effect on the cause. The endocrine glands play a vast role in brain chemistry. They play the primary role in the maintenance of its normal function. In fact, these glands directly control the metabolism of brain and nerve cells. Thus, any treatment for mental diseases which neglects this issue of endocrine involvement is of little if any consequence.

The majority of symptoms of mental diseases are also, incredibly, precisely the symptoms seen in glandular disorders. For instance, in hypothyroidism depression is perhaps the key presenting symptom, while panic attacks are a significant symptom of impaired adrenal function. Compulsive behavior, for which countless prescriptions of psychotropic drugs are dispensed, is another dominating symptom: it tells of adrenal exhaustion. Also, anxiety is largely a sign of adrenal dysfunction, while sluggish mental function is common in the thyroid type, as is poor memory and poor concentration. Also, according to Tintera poor concentration is the most common symptom of severe adrenal exhaustion, even more common than fatigue.

In testicular dysfunction anger and hostility dominate, while regarding ovarian disorders there is commonly depression, irritability, panic attacks, hot flashes, menstrual cramps, pelvic pain, breast disorders, and nervousness. All these symptoms may be diagnosed as mental disease. Yet, by no means are they primarily mental, rather, they are glandular. So, then, it is crucial for people who are suffering from such disorders to determine their body types. As a result, the cure can be achieved, while disasters are avoided.

The connection is definite. For instance, consider panic attacks. This disorder afflicts millions of Americans, primarily women. Routinely, doctors presume it is psychological. Yet, they fail to take into account the role of nutrition and/or diet. They completely neglect to make the endocrine connection, which is paramount. Panic attacks are largely related to blood sugar disorders. They are also related to an inability to cope. A kind of claustrophobic tendency can also provoke them, but this, too, is related to the coping mechanism. Bizarre smells and excessive noise, as well as tremendous stress, can provoke these attacks. Yet, all these functions are directly controlled by the adrenal glands. So, if the adrenal glands are strong, then, all such symptoms disappear.

Panic attacks are largely related to faulty adrenal function as well as imbalances in the entire endocrine system. The fact that women are the primary victims of this condition suggests a role for female hormones. Thus, if the ovaries are dysfunctional, these attacks may result. Thus, ideally, a treatment plan for panic attacks includes balancing these glands. This can be achieved with natural hormonal support. A natural ovarian formula containing wild kelp, undiluted royal jelly, wild sage, fennel, and fenugreek is ideal. Regardless, anyone who frequently suffers from panic attacks is likely adrenal body type. Such a person is also likely a sugar addict.

The role played by the ovaries in nervous disorders may explain an interesting phenomenon. In the military due to their tendency for claustrophobia-related panic attacks women are never commissioned to submarines. Yet, if foods or supplements specific for strengthening glandular function are given to such individuals, surely, they could withstand claustrophobic environments. Plus, invariably, with such therapy the panic attacks are eliminated.

So, for any mental disease it is crucial to determine the body type. This is more important than seeing a psychiatrist. What's more, it is surely more important than taking potent mood-altering drugs. For instance, in chronic depression thyroid and thyroid-adrenal types predominate. Manic depressive syndrome may also be a manifestation of sluggish thyroid. Retardation is also most commonly seen in thyroid types. Panic attacks are usually found in adrenal and thyroid-adrenal types as well as pituitary types. Most people with anxiety are adrenal and thyroid-adrenal. These are general rules. The point is the person should determine the specific type before submitting to medical therapies, which usually fail to treat the cause.

Even so, the first issue to consider in mental diseases is the condition of the hormone system. Of course, another serious consideration is the diet. By correcting any hormonal imbalances and improving the diet dramatic changes can be expected. With thyroid imbalances there is a depression of brain cell activity. With adrenal disorders the flow of blood and the utilization of glucose to the brain is disturbed. In the event of pituitary disorders there is usually inflammation in the brain as well as swelling. There may also be a disruption in the synthesis of neurotransmitters.

The brain is an end organ. It is dependent upon various substances for activating its chemistry. These substances are mainly the hormones, particularly thyroid hormone and adrenal hormones, but also pre-hormone substances such as serotonin and GABA. Without these various brain activating chemicals, this organ is essentially useless. Also, the vitamins D and B_{12} dramatically affect brain chemistry, and the former is, in fact, a hormone.

Malnutrition: the plague of modern humanity

That's right, Western people are malnourished. In other words, malnutrition is not just a disease of the poor or primitive. It is due to the intake of highly processed foods. It is also related to the nature of farming, that is the loss of top soil and the aggressive use of synthetic chemicals, which devastate the soil.

Malnutrition devastates the endocrine glands. These glands have a fast metabolic rate, so they consume a vast amount of nutrients. It also has harsh effects upon the brain. Here, a lack of nutrients can dramatically affect mood and, ultimately, may even cause severe neurological diseases.

All organs are dependent upon a steady supply of key nutrients: vitamins, minerals, fatty acids, and amino acids. Incredibly, if these organs are lacking even a single nutrient, they can be disabled. Yet, Americans are highly malnourished, lacking in multiple nutrients. Again, this is largely due to extensive consumption of processed foods. The processed foods rob nutrients. Plus, they lack the nutrients needed by the body to replenish the needs of the organs. Also, keep in mind that drugs destroy nutrients. Stress also robs the body of key substances, particularly trace minerals and vitamin C.

So, malnutrition is not just a disease of the poor nations. Rather, it is a plague of all Western civilization. Yet, how could this be? For instance, America and Britain are among the richest nations of the world. Even so, here the majority of the foods available are heavily processed and, in fact, adulterated. Purely natural foods grown on rich organic soil are relatively rare. Through the food processors a vast hoax has been perpetrated upon the people. This is because processed foods are the most nutritionally unfit foods in the world.

After World War II the truth about toxic foods was brought to the fore. Previously, false advertising had convinced the public that there was no harm in eating devitalized foods, including white sugar, flour, and rice. The truth was beginning to be revealed: white flour and sugar and the various foods made from them were the cause of the most dangerous diseases known. This was despite the fact that the food processors made outrageous claims, for instance, that white bread was nutritious, even a body builder, and that white sugar provided needed energy.

During the 1950s and 1960s the federal government, spurred by compelling research, prohibited such false claims. Researchers found that these substances destroyed tissues, never aiding them. Yet, this was merely a temporary compromise. No effort was made to forge an improvement in the food supply. Thus, the food giants were given unbridled ability to sell their goods, despite the known fact that they ultimately cause disease.

Processed foods cause a greater amount of disease than any other factor. This is proven by the fact that the elimination of such foods from the diet results in a rapid and dramatic improvement in health. Enter the endocrine glands, which are unable to function adequately on a processed food diet. In fact, the entire shape and appearance of the body can be distorted through the intake of such foods, which demonstrates the dramatic and derogatory effect of these foods upon the body. They even issue warnings about herbs, while saying nothing about poisonous foods and food additives. Incredibly, government agencies attempt to regulate mere herbs which have been used for thousands of years and which have never been proven to cause human harm. In contrast, such agencies do nothing to warn the public about known poisons such as MSG, sulfites, sucralose, fructose, corn syrup, refined sugar, and artificial colorings. These agencies perpetuate disease-causing foods and additives and work to crush all that is safe and perhaps curative.

The endocrine glands largely control the body's resistance to disease. They are also involved in life span, that is a strong endocrine system is perhaps the best defense against premature aging as well as death. How the body is nourished directly impacts the health. The glands are dependent upon adequate nourishment. If the food is entirely natural and if the proper types of foods are eaten, the glands are strengthened. If the food is depleted and/or processed, adulterated with chemical additives, sugar, corn syrup, corn starch, and white flour, the glands are rapidly weakened. Also, if the food is genetically engineered, as is the case with the majority of food in America, this devastates the glands. As a result, the ability of the body to cope with stresses is compromised. This is both physical and mental stress. The individual becomes vulnerable to sudden illnesses; however, the greatest debacle is that the development of chronic disease is assured. What a person eats directly impacts the health of the glands. A person should be cautious of the food consumed. Surely, at a minimum the labels must be carefully scrutinized for poisonous ingredients.

Hives and rashes, as well as inflammation in the throat, mouth, or tongue, as well as stomach disorders, intestinal disorders, and weakness of the immune system: all are symptoms that may be directly related to food which is consumed. Moreover, these symptoms and conditions are often the consequence of the consumption of genetically engineered foods. This is why the recipes in this book are free of GMOs. It is also why a source for pure non-GM foods is offered on the internet.

Regardless of what is consumed be sure these foods are nourishing to the glands. This is the ideal approach for achieving optimal health and for resisting the onset of degenerative disease.

The degree of malnutrition among North Americans is beyond comprehension. Quigley notes in his book *The National Malnutrition* that 999 out of every 1000 are severely deficient in key nutrients. Through surveys conducted in the 1940s and 1950s, he proved this fact. Think about the status today. All people are profoundly deficient, while a high percentage are incomprehensibly deficient. This is why there is virtually no one who is in perfect health. In other words, in the event of deficiency body functions will fail. Thus, it is easy to comprehend the dire state of affairs. The fact is today it seems that all people complain of certain health issues. If the nutritional and hormonal imbalances were corrected, a majority of these symptoms and/or health issues would also be corrected.

The key to optimal health is to be sure the cells get the nutrients they need. This can be accomplished through the consumption of high-nutrient foods, including animal products, plus food concentrates such as rice bran, oat bran, royal jelly, wild-source essential oils, crude cold-pressed nut/seed oils, wild raw greens extracts, wild raw berries extracts, and crude red grape powder. Only such quality concentrates, which are completely natural and chemical free, must be used. Such concentrates, as mentioned here, are also never genetically engineered.

Other excellent sources of concentrated nutrition are organic nuts/seeds, avocados, organic meat, organic poultry, whole organic eggs, and whole organic or raw milk products. These nutrient-dense foods/concentrates should be regularly consumed in the weekly diet. In the case of severe deficiencies such food concentrates should be consumed in large amounts. This is a natural and safe way to correct nutritional deficiencies. This is because food concentrates provide dense supplies of naturally-occurring vitamins, enzymes, and minerals, the kind the body is designed to use. As a result, overall health will improve. The hormone system will be vitalized. Cell function will normalize. Plus, diseases will be eradicated.

With the hormone typing system the results are spectacular. Often, they are virtually miraculous, as is demonstrated by the following case history:

Ms. R. is a 44-year-old woman, who could no longer care for herself. The victim of a surgery that went awry she was debilitated and had lost a great deal of weight, weighing under 75 pounds. She had lost her appetite and was extremely weak.

Endocrine assessment revealed she was adrenal type, and the appropriate treatment was begun, mainly crude emulsified paste of royal jelly (in a base of unprocessed raw pumpkinseed oil). Her improvement was remarkable. The appetite greatly improved, and quickly she began gaining weight. Within a month she was released and now lives a relatively normal life.

Chapter Eight
Toxins and Deficiencies

Once a person determines his/her endocrine type it is important to keep the body in top condition. The endocrine system is highly vulnerable to toxins and stress. Most poisons enter the body through the gut, and the endocrine system is highly sensitive to any noxious reaction in this region. One reason for this is the fact that many endocrine glands originated embryologically from the digestive tissues. So, these glands are inherently connected to the gut, for good reason.

The glands protect us. They must have an awareness of any threats to our systems. This is particularly true of the pituitary, thyroid, and pancreas, all of which are embryologically connected to the digestive tract. It is also true of the adrenal glands, which process all shock reactions as well as any exposure to poisons.

Everyone wants to be as healthy as possible. To achieve this it is necessary to protect the body from such toxins and stressors. This section will help the individual realize just what can poison this system as well as how to avoid it.

There are a number of substances which poison the glandular/metabolic system. The glands are highly vulnerable to the various effects of poisons. Fluoride is one of the most pervasive and destructive of these poisons. This substance has a direct and negative action on virtually all glands.

Anyone with a metabolic disorder could be suffering from fluoride poisoning. Children are readily poisoned, especially those suffering from impaired metabolism or disturbed mental function. Failure to thrive is another sign of metabolic poisoning. Metabolic poisons include refined sugar, heavy metals, aspartame, drugs, insecticides, herbicides, and perhaps the most toxic poison of all, fluoride.

A child who suddenly develops a heart defect or a thyroid disorder could be a victim of fluoride poisoning. Fluoride is an extreme intracellular poison. What's more, it has a predilection for the endocrine glands. Here, it can create enormous havoc, causing severe metabolic derangement as well as a host of diseases, including thyroid cysts, ovarian cysts, breast cysts, hypothyroidism, adrenal collapse, infertility, endometriosis, muscular diseases, and goiter. Notice the number of endocrine disorders on this list. Obviously, fluoride is a systemic poison, and, thus, it disrupts the entire endocrine chemistry. Its toxicity is due to its effects upon protein metabolism. It is particularly toxic to enzymes. In fact, it is capable of neutralizing enzyme activity. The enzymes are needed for the synthesis of endocrine hormones. Thus, it is crucial at all costs to avoid the exposure to and intake of such a poison.

All proteins are bound together by hydrogen bonds. Hydrogen is an atom similar in size to fluoride. Emsly and coworkers discovered that fluoride can displace hydrogen from proteins. When this occurs, the chemistry of the protein, whether biologically active, for instance, enzymes, or structural becomes disrupted. As a result, such proteins can no longer function normally. When proteins are damaged in this manner, a wide range of disorders result.

The incredible toxicity of fluoride against cellular proteins is perhaps best described by Drs. Froede and Wilson of the University of Colorado, who state that this poison destroys enzymes "by breaking and reforming hydrogen bonds." There is yet another mechanism: disruption of thyroid function. This toxicity was utilized by the medical profession. Incredibly, in what was certainly one of the most barbaric therapies in history in the early 1900s medical doctors prescribed fluoride to disable hyperactive thyroids. Because of the extreme toxicity, which led to numerous deaths directly due to fluoride poisoning, the practice was ultimately abandoned.

Fluoride is supremely toxic to human cells. According to Dr. Yiamouyiannis in his book *Fluoride: the Aging Factor* as little as 5 mg, the amount that most people consume daily by drinking fluoridated water, is enough to diminish thyroid activity. Fluoride's specific toxicity is related to the fact that, chemically, it is similar to iodine. Thus, it takes the place of iodine within critical molecules such as thyroid hormone. It does so in a manner that is known biochemically as irreversible, which means it creates for itself a permanent position. In other words, it completely blocks iodine's ability to function. As a result, the available amount of active or iodine-rich thyroid hormone declines significantly. The fact is excessive intake of fluoride can virtually halt the thyroid function, obliterating all hormone synthesis.

Fluoride is a categorical poison. It must never be consumed. Contrary to popular belief even the levels found in public drinking water are harmful. Once ingested, this poison is difficult to remove. It attaches aggressively to various proteins, as a molecular super-glue, binding up critical substances. There is no means for the body to remove it. Therefore, any amount is toxic.

Water is the primary source of this toxin, that is artificially fluoridated public water. Other primary sources include toothpaste (which should never be swallowed), fluoride-based rinses and mouthwashes, multiple vitamins (for infants and children), commercial food, beverages made with fluoridated water, commercial baby food, and fertilizer dust. For those who give their children commercial multiple vitamins be sure to read labels. Hundreds of infants and children have been poisoned every year as a result of fluoride-containing multiple vitamins. Fluoride–based rinses and toothpaste are also a major cause of such poisons. Avoid fluoride like the plague. Check the internet. Find sources of fluoride exposure. Then, systematically avoid it.

Allergic reactions: how they disrupt adrenal function

Allergic reactions poison the endocrine glands. This is largely because such glands must always deal with allergic reactions. In other words, they must process all such reactions. Thus, constant processing of allergic toxicity depletes endocrine strength.

Allergists who practice alternative medicine know that the constant exposure to allergenic substances depletes endocrine reserve. This may be manifested by vulnerability to hives, shock reactions, itchiness, digestive disorders, sore throat, bronchitis, asthma, and migraine headaches.

Exposure to allergenic, that is allergy-causing, substances leads to depletion of immune reserves. This also disrupts glandular function. The adrenal glands suffer the brunt of the damage. This is because these glands must deal with the inflammation that results from allergic reactions. Also, adrenal hormones are needed to calm the immune system, so it doesn't over-react. The thyroid gland and pituitary are also involved in reversing allergic toxicity. Regarding the pituitary this gland can swell dramatically after exposure to allergy-causing foods or chemicals. When allergenic foods or inhalants are avoided, the endocrine system gradually recovers. Thus, if a person continuously bombards his or her body with, for instance, allergenic foods, the glands are significantly weakened.

Allergy testing: is it necessary?

People are aware of the existence of inhalation allergies such as reactions to dust, dander, pollen, and mites. What is less well appreciated is that the most common ones which cause toxicity are the food allergies. A huge percentage of Western people, especially those who are chronically ill, suffer from food allergies. Illnesses and symptoms which are due to food allergies or intolerances include migraines, gallbladder attacks, colitis attacks, constipation, diarrhea, sinusitis, bronchitis, hives, depression, anxiety, seizures, arthritis, cystitis, and eczema to name a few. Elimination of all food intolerances leads to an improvement and even reversal of all such disorders. Thus, accurate tests for any unknown food intolerances may prove invaluable.

Ideally, in the construction of any diet plan allergenic foods should be discovered and eliminated. Each individual has had his/her pattern or allergies. Without testing there is no sure way to know these allergies. Yet, this poses a dilemma, because the availability of such testing is limited.

The majority of allergy tests available for foods are inaccurate. With inaccurate tests it is better not to get tested than to have misleading information. One test that is highly accurate is the Food Intolerance Test. This is a highly specialized test, the most accurate available. It is based on a kind of immunity known as cell mediated immunity. This test is only performed in one lab in the world. For more information regarding this test contact:

Food Intolerance Test
Continental Towers II
1701Golf Rd Suite 206
Rolling Meadows, Illinois 60008
1-847-640-1377
director@biotrition.com

For those who are unable to do such testing there are a number of other options. Surely, one of the easiest solutions is to simply avoid all highly poisonous food. This will dramatically reduce the tendency for allergy. In particular, all stimulants and food additives must be avoided. This alone will reduce the allergic tendency massively. Potentially toxic food components, such as cola bean, coffee bean, cocoa bean, MSG, sulfites, and NutraSweet, should be completely avoided. What's more, adrenal types should never consume coffee or black tea. Nor should they consume large amounts of chocolate (occasionally as a treat only). This is because of the stimulatory actions of these foods/beverages.

Such allergenic foods and chemicals must be avoided. This is because in the majority of people they cause great damage to the cells and organs and thus must be strictly avoided. When the immune system is exposed to such toxins, researchers have documented a telling finding. White blood cells explode and die on contact. This is proof that the regular consumption of highly allergenic foods is disasterous.

There are great benefits from eliminating allergenic foods. There is a simple tool for eliminating poisonous foods and food additives. This is by avoiding the major toxins and food additives. Also, in a research study, which was conducted on migraine patients, an interesting pattern of highly allergenic foods was discovered. These may be regarded as the top seven allergenic foods. So, if these foods, plus the chemicals/toxins, are avoided, this will suffice for most people. A list of the "must avoid" foods/chemicals includes:

Top seven foods

cheddar cheese
wheat
rye
sugar
Swiss cheese
barley and barley malt
corn and corn syrup

Chemicals/additives/stimulants

NutraSweet
cola
coffee bean
cocoa
black tea
sulfites
MSG
artificial flavors/colors
nitrates
saccharin
sucralose
baker's and brewer's yeast

If these foods/substances alone are eliminated, there will be a major improvement in overall health and much less stress on the endocrine system. Let the endocrine system be the source of stimulation. Never burden it with artificial stimulants, as well as consistent exposure to allergenic foods, which ultimately destroy it.

Through eliminating such toxins from the diet the endocrine glands are relieved. This will give the glands the most ideal opportunity to heal. To truly follow the appropriate plan for the endocrine type the recommended diet plus the knowledge of the food intolerance is ideal. If a person cannot achieve this, then simply follow the recommended diet for the type along with the elimination of the aforementioned foods, additives, and stimulants.

There are hundreds of symptoms of food allergies. There are also dozens of symptoms of inhalant allergies. All such reactions deplete endocrine reserve. Yet, food allergies are of far greater significance than many people realize. A variety of bothersome symptoms, as well as actual diseases, may be directly due to food allergies. Plus, the symptoms are rarely acute. So, people fail to realize the connection. This is why food allergy is known as the great mimicker. Symptoms which may be caused by food allergy include upset stomach, nausea, heartburn, gas, colitis attacks, intestinal cramps, bloating, hives, itchy rash, eczema, dermatitis, headaches, stiff neck, back pain, cracked skin, sinus pressure/drainage, sneezing fits, depression, irritability, palpitations, burping, burning eyes, itchy eyes, sties on the eyes, earaches, food cravings, runny nose, mood swings, swollen joints, pain in the joints, muscular pain, and dozens of others. Thus, it is readily apparent that food allergies cause great toxicity to the body. The endocrine glands bear the brunt of this damage. Therefore, in order to achieve total endocrine recovery the allergenic foods must be diagnosed and eliminated from the diet.

GMOs: accelerating the toxicity

The wide range of symptoms clearly demonstrates the toxicity caused by allergenic foods. Such a list of symptoms leaves no doubt regarding the harsh affects from eating these foods. In some individuals the regular intake of potentially toxic foods can wreak havoc. In addition to the aforementioned chemicals GM soy, canola, corn, and cottonseed must now also be added to the list. The latter are just as poisonous if not more so as the chemicals. Yet, most of these engineered foods also contain synthetic chemicals. Thus, such foods massively disrupt endocrine function. This is why sudden death is a consequence of the ingestion of GMOs. This is largely due to adrenal collapse. Yet, then the government which encourages the sale of such poisons frets over the safety of herbs? The fraud in this is obvious for all to see.

These GMO-tainted and chemical-infested foods are highly destructive, many of them outright carcinogenic. Incredibly, tens of thousands of people are sickened every year as a result of the intake of such additives. What's more, many die, and the number is difficult to count, since death is often attributed to other causes. In certain people allergic reactions are sufficiently toxic to cause death. This is why the adrenal glands are called to the fore. These glands are the primary means of the body to reverse toxic or life-threatening insults. When a poison is ingested, it is the adrenals which attempt to neutralize it. Cortisone is poured out. If the adrenal glands are weak, it could be a disaster. Such a reaction can be even up to 10-fold or more greater as a result of the ingestion of genetically altered food.

The adrenal glands: the body's anti-toxin system

The power of the adrenal glands is extensively proven by science. It was Myers who found that these adrenal glands have incomprehensible anti-toxic powers. In the test tube he injected cobra venom into an emulsion of cholesterol-rich adrenal cortex tissue. The venom was completely neutralized. Lewis found that animals with intact or strong adrenal glands could handle up to ten times the dose of cobra venom than those with weaker glands. Another study was done with rats. Using morphine as a test agent the strong rats resisted its toxicity, handling 500 times the dose of the weaker rats. The researchers attributed this detoxification power to its rich source of steroids, that is cholesterol. This demonstrates the importance of the regeneration of the adrenal cortex as a means of defense. This is surely achieved through the lipid- and fat-rich diets prescribed in this book as well as key nutritional supplements such as whole raw maca extract, crude natural-source vitamin C, triple-source Wild SaltCaps, wild raw greens drops, wild raw eight berries drops, and undiluted 3x fortified royal jelly.

These cholesterol molecules themselves are antioxidants to neutralize poisonous chemicals, but they are also waxes, which adsorb or bind noxious substances. This action is especially powerful against those chemicals which are soluble in fat. What's more, it is cholesterol in the form of bile acids, which is the body's system for purging toxic substances. Cholesterol, as bile acids, binds to a wide range of dangerous chemicals, transporting them through the liver into the intestines for excretion. Here, the liver acts as a filter to trap and purge toxic chemicals. The liver, then, makes the bile to get rid of toxic compounds. Yet, this process is entirely dependent upon cholesterol. This is why people with adrenal body types who are chemically sensitive must consume cholesterol on a regular basis, often in large quantities.

Milk allergy: a serious challenge

Some individuals are highly allergic to milk and milk products. Allergies to butter, cheese, cottage cheese, and even yogurt are relatively common. As mentioned previously perhaps most common is allergic intolerance to certain aged cheeses, particularly cheddar and Swiss cheese. Such cheese contains the bacterial ferment, known as tyramine, which is highly poisonous. This poison is also found in red wine and largely accounts for its toxicity. Cow's milk allergy is also relatively common, afflicting as many as one of four people. In this instance despite its nutritional value it is best to avoid milk or any of its derivatives. In some instances sheep's or goat's milk products may be tolerated, yet, in the highly sensitive individual it may be necessary to eliminate all milk products.

Especially for those who are suffering from an illness, there are simple ways to determine any allergenic foods. The best method is the aforementioned Food Intolerance Test. Or, simply eliminate all milk products from the diet for a reasonable period, like a month or two. Then, reintroduce a favorite milk product. If there is a noticeable or violent reaction to this, then it may be advisable to eliminate all forms of milk products permanently. Symptoms of milk-related poisoning include itchy rash, hives, spastic colon, constipation, diarrhea, blood in the stools, lung congestion, sinus problems, spastic muscles, and arthritis.

There is a real debacle in avoiding milk products. This is vitamin deficiency. If milk products are eliminated entirely, what is there to replace them? There is a kind of green milk available. Highly concentrated, it is available as a one ounce bottle. Known as wild greens flush this is a potent wild green extract, which is rich in riboflavin, the key vitamin provided by milk products. About a tablespoon per day provides the amount of riboflavin found in nearly a cup of milk. There is also the Super-5-Greens, another wild greens formula, which is a beverage. Also concentrated, it is rich in naturally occurring potassium, sodium, protein, and riboflavin. This contains extracts of wild raspberry leaf, spring horsetail rush, wild thistle, and wild lettuce leaf. It is only available online at AmericanWildFoods.com. Such wild greens cleanse all parts of the tissues, including the stomach, intestines, liver, and colon.

These greens are a kind of vegetable milk. Therefore, in particular for vegans and vegetarians they are highly sustaining. Eggs can replace many of the nutrients, however, people who are allergic to milk products may also react to eggs. Thus, meat must be relied upon for balancing nutritional needs. Nut milks may also be of value. They can be made at home. Ultimately, in many cases it is probably not the milk that is toxic but, rather, what is done to it. Thus, the processing, adulteration, and chemical contamination of the milk renders it a poison.

American milk: supreme toxin

In the United States commercial milk is of particular concern. This is because it most likely contains residues of the highly toxic genetically engineered substance, bovine growth hormone. Made by Monsanto this is a known carcinogen. Milk which contains residues of this synthetic hormone is unfit for human consumption. The fact is the Monsanto Corporation was fully aware of the dangers of this substance, and yet as is typical of its reckless propensities, it marketed it regardless. As proof of its danger in Canada it is banned.

Monsanto is reckless. In its quest to dominate world market it wreaks havoc upon the globe. The company even pays cash bribes to achieve its plots. All people must boycott the products made by Monsanto. One such product is the herbicide Round-Up. No one should use such a product. Of course, another is American commercial milk products, that is unless such milk products are labeled "free of bovine growth hormone."

In Canada based upon Monsanto's own research bovine growth hormone was banned. Incredibly, the Canadian researcher, Shiv Chopara, who revealed the dangers of this hormone, was ostracized, rather, fired. He waged a campaign to reinstate his reputation and won. Thus, the American farmers are the ones who suffer the consequences of the use of this hormone. This is diminished market share (due to European and other boycotts) plus an inferior product that people specifically avoid. Monsanto and similar corporations have perpetrated great damage to the human race. No one wants American milk. This is because it is poisonous. In fact, as a result of the creation of GM food Monsanto is responsible for a number of deaths and various illnesses, including allergic toxicity, anaphylactic shock, as well as cancer.

An effort must be made to resist this tyranny. In fact, there is such an effort, and it is succeeding. In the United States two major supermarket chains, Albertson's and the highly progressive Publix, have banned Monsanto's hormone from their private label milk. Reward such companies by buying their products. Also, when shopping in their stores, commend them. If you do tolerate milk, organic is the only reasonable choice, that is unless the dairy can assure you that its milk products are free of growth hormones. Thus, obviously, for those suffering from endocrine imbalances, particularly the pituitary type, the intake of commercial or non-organic milk products is ill-advised. Consume them only when absolutely necessary. Rather, buy only from organic sources.

The so-called food products of Monsanto are endocrine poisons. These products must never be consumed. Such foods or rather poisons include commercial corn, canola oil, commercial soy, cottonseed meal and cottonseed oil, commercial milk (unless proven to be free of bovine growth hormone) and, of course, all products made from soy. No one should buy any of this company's products. These are all based upon corruption. In particular, Monsanto-corrupted milk is an extreme allergen as well as carcinogen. Again, people should boycott such milk products, that is until the marketplace responds by banning all bovine growth hormone-tainted milk. Does anyone want their innocent female relatives and friends to develop spontaneous breast cancers? This is a deliberate consequence of the regular ingestion of growth hormone-contaminated milk.

Infection and endocrine types: a critical factor

The body's many glands are highly vulnerable to infection. Few doctors appreciate how common such infection is. Virtually no doctor regards a disease of the glands as infective. However, commonly, the glands are infected in a kind of chronic way, without obvious symptoms. The infectious agents vary, but in general fungi, yeasts, bacteria, and viruses may all infect the endocrine glands.

A hint is given on autopsy. Using the adrenal glands as an example pathologists have discovered that as many as one in three people have an infection in these glands. The culprit is, incredibly, tuberculosis. The only symptom is usually fatigue, perhaps night sweats, and often mid- to lower-back pain. Yet, in people with chronic health problems what the pathologists failed to uncover is an equally dire agent: syphilis. This organism isn't 'seen.' Rather, it is inherited. In other words, if a parent or grandparent had this disease, the progeny can develop it. Like the TB bacteria, this germ thrives in biologically

280 The Body Shape Diet

active glands, and, thus, it readily infects the adrenal gland, thyroid, ovaries, and testes. Here, such germs find the nutrients they need to survive. Again, it is difficult to culture. However, its presence can be measured through a special machine. This technique is known as electrodermal testing and is similar to the principles of kinesiology. Otherwise, it nearly always goes undetected, but the chronic disability it causes can be devastating.

Again, people don't normally think of the glands as being infected. Yet, the glands are equally as vulnerable to infection as any other tissue, perhaps more so. So, with any glandular disorder infection must be considered. This is because of the high metabolic rate of these organs. There is plenty of oxygen and nutrients, and so, microbes thrive in such an environment. Plus, these glands concentrate nutrients, which the germs require for survival. Consider the mumps virus, which now only rarely infects people. It has a predilection for attacking the testes and/or ovaries. The candida yeast readily infects the thyroid, uterus, ovaries, and prostate, while TB settles mainly in the adrenals.

Also, a wide range of fungi readily infect the glands. Truss and others have documented the existence of a kind of systemic fungal infection, which attacks potentially any endocrine gland. This is caused by the notorious yeast *Candida albicans*. A significant portion of those diagnosed with thyroid and/or adrenal disorders may well suffer from such an infection, where the yeast fully inhabits the glands, causing extensive damage. Unless the yeast is eradicated, the disease will persist. The endocrine glands are greatly compromised from such a germ invasion. Thus, in order for improvement to occur—in order for function to be normalized—the germ must be eradicated.

This is achieved through the intake of wild spice extracts. These are potent substances for eradicating infections, even deep-seated ones such as those which occur in the glands. Interestingly, scripture, that is the Bible, deems wild spices, specifically oregano, as purging agents, which must be utilized. This is substantiated by modern research. A number of spices have been proven to be powerful germ killers, which can virtually purge any germ from the body.

Perhaps premier in this is the multiple spice complex. This is made from wild mountain-grown spices. Such spices, notably wild oregano, cumin, bay leaf, and sage, contain potent antiseptics, known as phenols. According to research at Georgetown Medical Center published in *Molecular and Cellular Biology, September 4, 2001,* multiple spice oils completely obliterated all traces of yeasts within living tissue. Within 30 days the yeasts, which in laboratory mice had caused systemic infection, were eradicated. A slow-release multiple spice complex is ideal, because it gradually releases in the colon, where the fungi and other pathogens live. Such a slow-release formula is emulsified in bees wax and, thus, is well tolerated, even by those with sensitive systems. This, combined with oil of wild oregano taken under the tongue, is an ideal purge. Other multiple spice complexes include capsules made from vacuum dried wild spice oils.

Yeasts are aggressive germs. They readily gain entrance to the organs, inhabiting them. The immune system has a difficult time destroying them. Plus, they tend to mutate in order to avoid extermination. Based on the latest scientific research spice extracts, particularly those made from the edible wild varieties, are a potent and reliable cure. Such extracts kill yeasts and other invaders on contact, plus they bolster the immune response against such invaders. A clinical evaluation in England proved that wild oregano alone in the form of Mediterranean steam-extract oil (in an extra virgin olive oil base) caused a significant improvement in humans with yeast-related chronic fatigue syndrome. Thus, the key natural medicines for eradicating these germs are Mediterranean wild spice oils.

So, again, adrenal types are usually infected with TB, perhaps syphilis or other spirochetes. These are chronic infections, not actively infective. They cannot transmit it to anyone, except, perhaps, as a kind of chronic disturbance (through sex). Again, much of the toxicity can be purged through the regular intake of wild spice oils such as the blue label wild oregano oil. Pituitary types are often infected by vaccine viruses, which contaminate the brain and, thus, the pituitary gland. Thyroid types are frequently infected by a wide range of fungi, as well as in some cases TB, especially those with chronic lung or bone disorders.

MSG: nerve toxin

Every effort should be made to avoid this toxin. There is no way a person can improve the endocrine system if this poison is regularly consumed. This is because MSG disrupts the nervous system and even directly intoxicates the glands. It also corrupts the higher centers, that is the hypothalamus, the pineal, and the pituitary, which control endocrine secretion.

MSG is the abbreviation for monosodium glutamate. This substance has no nutritional value and is, rather, a destroyer of nutrients. Thus, it is a corruption invented by the food processors. This is because it creates an addiction for processed foods. It does so by disrupting the flow of neurotransmitters in the brain.

Highly toxic, this chemical disrupts the nerve tissues, even causing nerve damage. Blaylock in his book *Excitotoxins* states categorically that MSG, if consumed for a prolonged enough period, causes brain damage.

Certainly, this substance is a major cause of allergic reactions. This alone is reason to avoid it. People with the adrenal type tend to react violently to it, as do those with the pituitary type.

Look for this substance on food labels. It may be readily disguised. On labels the terms MSG, monosodium glutamate, hydrolyzed vegetable protein, and autolyzed yeast are evidence for the use of the contaminant. Avoid foods containing MSG like the plague.

Sulfites: cellular poison

Sulfites are another common food additive which must be avoided. These toxins are essentially a dried form of sulfuric acid. They are totally synthetic. It is merely a way for chemical companies to create continuous profit. There is no need to add these chemicals to food. All they do is alter the color of the food. Essentially, they are an anti-browning agent. This is why they are so commonly used in French fries. Also, they are used to preserve processed fruit.

Sulfite allergy is common. These chemicals are a major cause of asthma attacks. In some people their ingestion readily causes hives. Furthermore, every year sulfites cause several dozen deaths in the United States, usually due to sudden allergic shock.

Completely avoid the ingestion of sulfites. These are found listed on labels as sulfites, sodium bisulfite, sodium sulfite, and sodium metabisulfite. These toxins disrupt the entire endocrine system, while also poisoning the immune system. They are so poisonous that they may cause immediate toxicity in the form of shortness of breath or asthma attacks, hives, or circulatory collapse. Thus, the ingestion of these toxins must be strictly prohibited.

Chapter Nine

The Right Metabolic Diet

It is critical to eat based upon metabolism. This is because metabolism is the basis of life. For instance, to level their blood sugar adrenal types must eat fat and salt, to balance their energy and speed metabolism thyroid types must eat protein, particularly animal protein, plus cooked vegetables and raw salads, and to balance their delicate metabolism pituitary types ideally eat lean game, fish, seafood, and foods rich in essential fatty acids, along with berries and salads. Food directly impacts the glands' functions, either aiding them or disrupting them. The way the body metabolizes food has everything to do with food selection, but it is also controlled by the person's metabolic type. Obviously, if a person is unable to metabolize starch, they shouldn't eat it. If another person cannot process sugar, then this must be avoided. If another person has difficulty digesting heavy fats—such as the pituitary type—then, these must be restricted.

If the metabolism is slow, for instance, as is seen in thyroid and pituitary types, then, regardless of the individual the consumption of starchy foods must be curbed. Rather than potatoes, peas, corn, grains, and rice one should eat dark green leafy vegetables, cruciferous vegetables (cooked), organic meat, organic organ meats, whole organic eggs, and nuts and seeds. Wild rice, a seed, could be a starch source. Plus, for true thyroid types cruciferous vegetables should never be eaten raw but, rather, should be cooked or steamed. For pituitary types alternative grains, such as amaranth, quinoa, and teff, are ideal; they are higher in protein than commercial grains and are more readily digested.

If the metabolism is medium to fast—such as is the case with many of the adrenal types—then, a certain amount of starch can be healthy, as is the sugar of fruit. These are general rules. There are also specific issues, for instance, the need in pituitary types for large amounts of omega-3s and vitamin E as well as thyroid types. Regarding vitamin E the best and safest type is that extracted from sunflower seeds, ideally emulsified in a base of crude pumpkinseed and wild red palm oils. For pituitary types, who are highly sensitive, it is particularly important only to use this type.

The muscular type has a medium metabolism. To stay lean and muscular such a type must eat goodly amounts of protein and vegetables. For energy fruit and raw honey are ideal. Here, too, starches must be consumed moderately. For muscular types while starches can be consumed and form a valuable source of energy, fruit and raw honey are superior, and they are certainly superior to wheat, rye, corn, and oats. Regardless, the proteins in the latter foods are incomplete and, thus, are incapable of supporting the demands of their muscular systems. Yet, when they are active, muscular types can handle larger amounts of starch than any other. However, for those who are sedentary, such starches act as metabolic poisons.

So, the diet must be based upon the following: whether the person is a thyroid, adrenal, thyroid-adrenal, adrenal-thyroid, or pituitary type, or, if these are not definitive, whether a person is a thyroid-muscular or pituitary-thyroid-adrenal. This is the starting point. True, there is much interest in the blood type diet. This also has value. Yet, it is best to begin with the metabolic type and use the blood type for supplemental information, because the metabolism plays a greater role in determining food intake than the blood type.

The basic plan

What follows is the basic diet for each endocrine type. For more information see the recipe section, which lists specific recommendations for each type.

Thyroid type (slow to medium metabolizer)

Diet should emphasize animal protein, all from organic sources. There is no restriction on such protein. Protein-rich foods can be eaten with every meal. Pork is prohibited. Fruit is to be consumed in moderation. This type should eat large amounts of salad greens. Cruciferous vegetables are allowed, but must be cooked to destroy any anti-thyroid factors. Tomatoes and avocados are ideal. Olives and olive oil are also ideal, along with avocado oil and crude, unprocessed, dark pumpkinseed oil. Sacha inchi oil may also be consumed. This is most nutritionally complete of all plant-source omega-3 fatty acid supplements. What's more, for those with thyroid-related weight gain the omega 3 fatty acids in sacha inchi oil help speed the burning of fat. For thyroid types this is only needed in modest quantities such as a tablespoon daily.

Nuts and seeds must be consumed in moderation. Again, animal food must be emphasized, along with vegetation. Remote-source kelp and sea vegetables are valuable. Seafood is particularly ideal, because it is rich in salts and natural iodine, which are much needed by the thyroid. Alternative grains which are acceptable include teff, quinoa, and amaranth. Food that is difficult to metabolize, namely grains, refined sugar, sweets, and chocolate, should be avoided. Potatoes can be eaten occasionally (with the skin on), but squash is preferable. It is best to scrape out the starchy part of the potato, and eat only the skin. Rice bran/polish concentrates are invaluable. Such concentrates must be consumed on a daily basis to provide a dense supply of the necessary B vitamins (Note: a purely whole food-based B complex supplement is now available made from concentrates of rice bran, torula yeast, and royal jelly).

It must be emphasized that this is a truly low carbohydrate diet. Many thyroid types can be exceedingly slow metabolizers. They deserve the distinction of super-slow metabolizers. They simply cannot process sugar and starch into energy. Thus, the excessive intake of such substances, in fact, even the most modest intake, greatly disrupts body chemistry. Surely, these types can never eat refined flour products or white sugar nor any foods made from such substances. That would truly be devastating. In fact, a diet high in white flour and sugar, along with well done meat, largely causes thyroid disorders. White flour and sugar destroy key nutrients needed by the thyroid for metabolism. In addition, they are devoid of any nutrients. This is why the intake of such foods is so devastating. For proper metabolism the thyroid type needs key nutrients, particularly thiamine, riboflavin, pyridoxine, pantothenic acid, magnesium, and zinc. The thyroid gland needs the essential amino acid tyrosine. All such nutrients are destroyed by white flour and white sugar.

It is important to hold to this diet and never deviate. Never eat horrible food. This is the only way the person will regain true health. The body needs nutrients for combustion. In other words, the normal metabolic rate is dependent upon readily available nutrients, needed for burning the food that is consumed into energy. If any of these nutrients are missing, then the burning mechanism is disabled.

It is also important to reiterate the danger of grains in general. Again, for the thyroid type the metabolic rate is exceedingly slow. This means that the digestive juices are poorly produced. There is a reduction in the efficiency of all the digestive organs: the stomach, intestines, liver, gallbladder, and pancreas. Even the function of the colon is impaired. Thus, difficult-to-digest foods, such as gluten-containing grains—wheat, rye, oats, and barley— are prohibited. They are tough to digest, even for people with normal digestion. Thus, for the sluggish metabolizers their consumption is catastrophic. The point is, again, there is no way these sluggish metabolizers can make sufficient digestive juices to completely digest grains. Easier-to-digest starches are preferable, notably wild rice, rice bran, sweet potato (mainly the skin and the first layer under it), yacon, and rice polish, as well as amaranth and teff. Even so, the diet must be mostly meat, eggs, milk products, and vegetables. For the thyroid type a perfect meal is a large salad with feta cheese, topped with a few pine nuts and plenty of oil and vinegar.

Thyroid-adrenal type (medium metabolizer)

Fatty foods are acceptable, as are animal proteins. Fruit is superior to vegetables. Whole grains in moderation are acceptable, but be wary of wheat. Salads are an ideal food, topped with high quality omega 3-rich vegetable oils, such as sacha inchi oil, sesame oil, and/or pumpkinseed oil, and feta cheese. Heavy oils, such as remote-source poppy seed oil, crude cold-pressed pumpkinseed oil, and extra virgin olive oil, should also be consumed. Fish and seafood are excellent foods. However, due to issues of contamination they must be consumed in moderation. In this type red meat and wild game can be eaten in quantity. The ideal type of oils to consume are a combination of those rich in saturated fat, such as butter, and those rich in monounsaturates and/or omega-3s such as extra virgin olive oil, wild sockeye salmon oil, and the aforementioned.

Adrenal (all ranges of metabolism, but often medium-to-fast)

In this type a wider variety of foods is consumed. Fatty- and protein-rich food can be combined with starchy ones. Fruit is superior to vegetables. All sorts of fats should be consumed, especially those rich in cholesterol. Ideal foods include whole organic eggs, whole milk products, including cheese, fatty meats, avocados, olives, fatty fish, lobster, and crab. Excessive amounts of vegetables should be avoided. The person may actually dislike them. Instead, fruit should be eaten, especially tomatoes, olives, avocados, and berries. Also, kiwi, papaya, sour oranges, lemons, limes, grapefruit, and melon are acceptable, but these should be salted. Even so, people with this type should never eat excessive amounts of melon, just a wedge or two occasionally. This is because melon is too high in potassium. However, the high potassium content can be neutralized by the liberal use of salt. Lamb is a particularly good food, as is turkey with the skin on. Nuts are acceptable in moderation, especially salted. If not salted, be sure to add salt.

Fruit should ideally be balanced with protein or fat such as cheese, yogurt, whole milk, or meat. Or, the fruit can be eaten with nuts. Maca concentrate and yacon syrup are also invaluable, as is, of course, royal jelly.

The best starches to consume are boiled potato, baked or raw sweet potato, wild rice, and brown rice. Rice crackers are an ideal snack. Some whole grains may also be tolerated.

Pituitary (super-slow metabolizer)

People with this type must avoid heavy greasy food. They may eat modest amounts of animal foods, but they must make sure they are lean. If relatively unpolluted fish is available, this should be a focus. Bison is the ideal meat (see Americanwildfoods.com). Also, organic organ meats are ideal: liver, tongue, sweetbreads, and kidneys. Nuts and seeds are fine in moderation. Nut and seed oils should be consumed, focusing on sacha inchi oil, crude pumpkinseed oil, crude cold-pressed black seed oil, and crude cold-pressed sesame oil (Turkish source only). Wild greens should be consumed as often as possible, either as food or as supplements (the greens flushing drops or the wild Super-5-

Greens, as found on the internet). These wild greens extracts should be taken ideally on a daily basis. Fruit is also well tolerated but must be relatively low in sugar. The best fruits for this type are blueberries, strawberries, cranberries, raspberries, blackberries, and currants. Melon is also ideal and should be salted. Pears and sour apples may also be well tolerated; these must be salted. Sea vegetables may also be a boon for this type. Berry concentrates are also ideal, such as the high-grade wild eight berries drops and the Mediterranean pomegranate concentrate.

The consumption of salads must be liberal. The salads must be topped with nuts and seeds, while smothered in essential fatty acid-rich oils such as organically grown sacha inchi oil, cold-pressed avocado oil, and crude unprocessed dark pumpkinseed oil. Other recommendations are found in the recipe section.

When the oils are used as a salad dressing, they must be consumed. The drippings should never be wasted in the bowl. This is where all the nutrients settle. It is certainly acceptable to also add a fine vinegar or lemon juice, along with the omega-3-rich oils such as the organic sacha inchi oil. This is a tasty and healthy way to enjoy salads.

Chapter Ten

Endocrine-Boosting Recipes

Now, it is time to enjoy. There are recipes for all the body types. Some recipes are ideal for all types, others specific types. All that is necessary is to select any of the recipes and build menus. Meals can be created based upon these choices. Included are various recipes, nutrient-rich shakes, smoothies, and foods, which will boost endocrine health. Or, based upon the knowledge in this book make up your own recipes.

Special nutrients or additives are included for each type. However, many of the recipes can be used interchangeably. For instance, most thyroid types will do well with the pituitary recipes and visa versa. The pituitary recipes are to a degree good for any category, since this gland helps stimulate the function of all others.

Adrenal types require a unique approach. While each adrenal person is unique, here, the food is often fat-rich. It is even rich in fat drippings and fatty skin. For the adrenal type there is no need to trim the fat off the meat. Plus, when roasting meat the drippings must be consumed. Pour them back over the meat, even the vegetables.

Adrenal and thyroid-adrenal types will thrive on this. For these types salt is a food. Incredibly, here excess potassium acts as a poison, while salt causes the person to thrive. Thus, for adrenal types potassium-rich salt substitutes are completely banned.

Thyroid types also need salts. However, they need primarily the tissue salts found in, for instance, deep sea fish, seafood, and red meat. Even so, they may liberally use sea salt on any meat dish. For thyroid types the meat need not be lean. Soup should ideally include seafood and kelp or at least chunks of organic meat.

The pituitary type also has special needs. These needs are a combination of the needs found in both the adrenal and thyroid types. In particular, recipes for this type are relatively low in carbohydrate. In this body type any carbohydrate has the tendency to be converted to fat. However, the safest type of carbohydrate is fruit. Thus, relatively low sugar fruits are included in these menus, while most starches are excluded.

Compared to starch fruit is easy to metabolize. In fact, in some instances fruit stimulates the metabolic rate. This is particularly true of wild berries or their raw extracts. So, it is better for pituitary types to eat fruit as a snack rather than grains. A bowl of fruit is infinitely superior to a roll, croissant, or muffin.

Pituitary types thrive on essential fatty acids. However, these must be the right type. Excess saturated fat disturbs essential fatty acid metabolism. Thus, when cooking meat, pituitary types must be sure to trim all visible fat. Plus, fat digestion is usually sluggish with this type. Foods rich in essential fatty acids are the focus. People with this type suffer from an inordinately slow metabolism. This also explains the emphasis in these menus on the use of special kinds of seed oils, which are rich in essential fatty acids. These oils include crude fortified pumpkinseed oil, poppyseed oil, and organically grown sacha inchi oil. These are highly digestible and speed the metabolic rate.

The ideal essential fatty acids are the various omega-3s, either from fish or vegetable sources. This is also why wild game, rich in omega-3s, is more ideal for this type than commercial meats, the latter being rich in saturated fats. Zinc is also needed by the pituitary. This is why the diet must contain a certain amount of animal foods, since animal foods, such as red meat and eggs, are the top dietary source of this nutrient. This is also why the diet must be low in commercial grains, since, for instance, wheat, rye, and oats destroy zinc.

Instead of creamy or greasy foods they should feast on nuts, seeds, and nut butters, wild berries and wild berry juices. The brans of grains, particularly rice and oat bran, are also acceptable.

The majority of pituitary types are Anglo-Saxons, although, increasingly, people of other races, for instance, blacks and hispanics who follow the typical Western diet are developing this syndrome. In the Mediterranean, as well as in those of Mediterranean ancestry, the thyroid type, as well as thyroid-adrenal type, predominate. Adrenal types are mainly found in people of Anglo-Saxon descent, although increasingly people of Asian descent, as they more thoroughly adopt a Western-style diet, are developing it.

The pituitary is highly sensitive to fatty acid nutrition. Thus, if this nutrition is disturbed, so is this gland's function. In fact, with the wrong fatty acids it becomes inflamed. This is why the intake of the appropriate essential fatty acids is crucial. Plus, to achieve the most spectacular results the intake must be consistent until metabolism normalizes. The thyroid also has a high need for essential fatty acids, but not as great as the pituitary. The adrenals have a lesser need and are more dependent upon saturated fats and, particularly, lipids, that is cholesterol. In fact, regarding the adrenals essential fatty acids, particularly the omega-6 types and even some omega-3s, are too aggressive and may actually compromise adrenal function. In excess they actually oxidize adrenal hormones and deplete adrenal steroid reserve. Incredibly, the right metabolic diet is for each type based largely upon fatty acid nutrition.

So, for adrenal types the diet is high in saturated fat, monounsaturates, and cholesterol and relatively low in unsaturates. Regarding vegetable oils the best ones are wild red palm oil, extra virgin olive oil, crude cold-pressed pumpkinseed oil, cold-pressed sesame oil, and similar heavy/nutritious oils. In pituitary types the best oils are those which are lighter, that is higher in omega-3s, such as organically grown sacha inchi oil, berry seed essential fatty acids, and crude cold-pressed pumpkinseed oil, as well as, unrefined fish oils, particularly fatty wild sockeye salmon oil. For thyroid types the best oils are a combination of extra virgin olive oil, some red palm oil, pumpkinseed oil, virgin coconut oil, and a certain amount of sacha inchi oil. Regardless, all these oils are healthy and may be used to a degree by all types. Thyroid types should avoid flaxseed oil, because it is too high in goitrogens. However, they can occasionally consume ground flaxseed, especially if it is toasted. Adrenal types will likely discover that if they regularly consume huge amounts of essential fatty acids, particularly flaxseed oil, it tires them and may even cause inflammation.

People with thyroid types who suffer from weight gain on the front of the body also have slow metabolism. In this case the intake of omega-3s should be high.

The effort to include fatty fish in the diet is now compromised. This is due to the dilemma of pollution. Now, a person must limit the intake of these fish. This is because large ocean fish are heavily contaminated, particularly with mercury as well as PCBs. These fish include halibut, tuna, bluefish, and salmon and can be consumed on a limited basis, about three or less servings per month. In this regard it has been determined that canned tuna is lower in mercury than fresh tuna. Sardines and herring can be consumed more frequently, like once or twice per week. In particular, king mackerel, swordfish, and marlin must be strictly avoided. Even so, for any fish eater adjustments must be made to cleanse contaminants. This can be accomplished through the intake of a raw wild greens flush and/or the super wild greens juice as a natural purging agent. Also, a purge made from a combination of wild raw greens, spice oils, vinegar, and cold-pressed oils is effective. Thus, whenever eating questionable fish take both the purge and the wild raw greens drops.

Incredibly, essentially, the human being has made the food from the oceans—that once pristine realm—unfit for human consumption. This is why the more pure and uncompromised organically grown sacha inchi oil, a truly

'Pure-Omega,' is the ideal source of omega-3s. There are no heavy metals in this oil. Another option is the high-grade unrefined wild sockeye salmon oil, which is exceedingly low in heavy metals compared to all other fatty fish sources.

There are a few rules which are helpful for selecting foods for each body type. In the thyroid type the metabolism is slow. So, excessive starch intake is counterproductive. Also, thyroid types often do poorly with grains, and, thus, the preferred starches are whole potatoes and brown rice. Wild rice is particularly ideal. Lower in starch than commercial rice this is a dense source of nutrients and can be freely added to the menu for all types. It is also a natural source of essential fatty acids, especially the truly wild remote-source variety. Other sources of natural essential fatty acids include fatty fish, the skin of poultry, wild game, seafood, dark greens, purslane, avocados, and nuts.

Again, the majority of such slow metabolizers are northern European in heritage. This heritage largely explains their vulnerability as well as their nearly complete intolerance to refined sugars and starches. This intolerance would be expected. They are relatively direct ancestors of the prehistoric Cro-Magnon man, a being who ate almost exclusively protein. This is far from a claim that, today, the thyroid and/or pituitary type must only eat meat. However, the emphasis is obvious, which is that protein, some fruit, raw honey as a sweetener (like meat, this was an ancestral food), and vegetables with only minimal grains, the latter consisting largely of the brans of grains, is the ideal diet for most people. For thyroid types nuts and seeds are also a part of the diet, but meat is more ideal. In contrast, refined potatoes, bread, cereals, and sweets must be avoided.

The recipes are a guide. Even so, use them to make your own recipes.

Regardless of the endocrine type relish this lovely food and enjoy. It is all rich and healthy. Plus, it is loaded in nutrients. Note: there are specialized supplements mentioned throughout the book, as well as unusual high-grade foods. Many of these specialized items are available at Americanwildfoods.com. This is a fine food site, since the majority of the items are remote-source, wild, and/or organic. What's more, they are all free of genetically engineered compounds (GMOs). Specialty items unavailable in traditional stores are capitalized. These items are available on the web and also in a few high quality health food stores.

The value of each recipe for the various metabolic types is identified. For each recipe the types that it is appropriate for are listed. Of course, many recipes are universal. Specialty items can be purchased on the internet, for instance, the Seggiano items, sour extract of pomegranate, maca, and red sour grape. Even so, for some of these items adequate substitutes may be found in higher quality health food stores. Again, all items listed in capitals are highly specialized foods.

A note on fluids: the hormones operate in a fluid environment. After meals, be sure to drink plenty of fluids. Do not drink large amounts of fluids with meals, as this dilutes the digestive secretions, which must be concentrated for ideal digestion.

The following recipes which are universal are listed with the distinction "all types." Enjoy both wonderful taste and fantastic health. That is the endocrine-metabolic body type guarantee.

Chapter Eleven

Recipes

Soups and Salads

Artichoke Soup (thyroid, muscular)

1 small head celery

1 turnip

1 onion

3 ounces butter

2 pounds artichokes

1 pint boiling organic milk

2½ quarts pure water

toasted pine nuts (few)

sea salt

Clean and slice vegetables and stew in saucepan in butter for half an hour. Wash and peel artichokes, cut in slices, and add with about one pint water to other vegetables. When those have stewed to a smooth pulp, put in the remainder of the water; simmer for 5 minutes and pass through a sieve. Return to saucepan, and add boiling milk slowly. Serve with toasted pine nuts.

Cheesy and Garlicky Cauliflower Soup (mainly adrenal but also thyroid)

Adrenal types do fairly well with cheese, especially if it is cooked. This is because cooking kills any molds on the cheese, to which such individuals are highly sensitive. The cheese also helps prevent a blood sugar rush from the potatoes. This is why cheese or sour cream should always be included with cooked potatoes.

1 medium potato, peeled and diced (makes about 2 cups when diced)

1 large cauliflower, broken or cut into small florettes

3 green onions, diced

2 cloves chopped garlic

2 tablespoons chopped leeks

1½ cups chopped onion

2 teaspoons sea salt

dash coriander

4 cups water

¾ cup whole organic milk

½ teaspoon caraway seeds

3 teaspoons fresh dill

2 cups grated organic Monterey Jack cheese, packed

green shoots of onion, diced (optional)

In a saucepan add potato, all but 2 cups cauliflower, garlic, leek, onion, salt, and water. Bring to a boil, then simmer until very tender. In a blender (or food processor) blend; transfer to a large pot or Dutch oven. Steam the remaining cauliflower until just tender; do not overcook. Add to puree with remaining ingredients. Warm gently and serve topped with extra cheese, dash coriander, and sprinkling of green shoots of onion.

Endocrine note: The salt and cheese offset the high amount of potassium and vegetable alkalines in the cauliflower. Thus, this is a balanced vegetable meal for the adrenal type.

B Vitamin-Rich Pine Nut Soup (all types)

4 ounces pine nuts

2 ounces finely minced onion

1 or 2 ounces organic butter

1 pint water

1 quart organic whole milk

1 ounce brown rice flour

2 teaspoons rice bran

Pulverize pine nuts; with mortar and pestle grind rice bran until fine. Fry with onion in saucepan in butter. Stir in brown rice flour and when well mixed, add water gradually; then, heat milk and add slowly, while mixing. Heat until well cooked and serve hot, topped with a few toasted pine nuts.

Strong Onion Soup with melted organic Swiss or Monterey Jack cheese (all types)

2 or 3 tablespoons butter (or extra virgin olive oil)

one large or two medium onions, thinly sliced

2 small to medium cloves garlic, minced

1 teaspoon Marmite (concentrated yeast extract), optional

2 teaspoons coarse unbleached sea salt

1 teaspoon arrowroot (to thicken soup)

1 tablespoon freshly grated horseradish

2 teaspoons dry mustard

2 cups water

1½ cups grated cheese

dash coriander or curry powder
dash paprika (for topping when done)
1½ cups warm whole/organic milk

In a pot or Dutch oven heat butter until melted. Add sliced onions, garlic, sea salt, and mustard; over medium heat cook for about 10 minutes or until onions are soft. Gradually sprinkle arrowroot, stirring as needed, then add Marmite: mix well. Add water and horseradish and stir; cook for about five additional minutes. Add cheese and milk; stir throughout with wooden spoon for several minutes or until smooth. Add remaining seasonings and top with dash paprika, as desired.

Endocrine note: To strengthen metabolism this onion soup serves as a hearty meal. The added horseradish and Marmite extract give it invigorating power. Eat this soup often, especially before an athletic event.

Simple Creamy Spinach Soup (thyroid, muscular)

enough organic spinach to make two cups of juice, well washed
pint whole organic milk (if you want this creamier, also add 3 T. heavy
    cream)
Herbamere or sea salt
handful pre-cooked wild rice (optional)

Simply heat all ingredients and serve; simple and fast. Do this with kale or chard.

Celery and Wild Rice Soup (all types)

1 stalk celery
2 large yellow onions
1 blade mace
12 peppercorns tied in a muslin bag

2 ounces True Hand-Picked Wild Rice (AmericanWildFoods.com)

2 T. almond butter (plus 1 T. oil from the top of the butter)

1 ounce brown rice flour

3 pints vegetable stock

1 teaspoonful sweet herb mix (or basil, parsley, chervil)

¼ pint whole organic milk or cream, warmed

sea salt as needed

In a large saucepan melt butter. Slice onions and celery, cutting into small pieces. Fry both in the nut butter and nut oil, without letting them brown. Add rice and 3 pints vegetable stock; stew until tender. Put in peppercorns and seasoning; cook for another ten minutes. Remove peppercorns and herbs, and then rub through sieve. Return to the saucepan, reheat, and add the milk or cream and rice flour gradually, just before serving.

Endocrine note: Celery is rich in sodium; this means it is good for the adrenals. So, this soup, while vegetable, is an adrenal tonic, but only if extra sea salt is added. Brown rice provides B vitamins. For added nutrition top this soup with a teaspoon of Organic Rice Bran.

Rich Tomato Soup (all types)

2 pounds organic tomatoes

2 large onions

2 ounces High-Grade Extra Virgin Olive Oil (Seggiano Brand)

2 ounces butter

12 allspice tied in muslin bag

½ teaspoonful dried basil

½ teaspoonful dried Wild Oregano from Bunches

1 quart pure water

1 ounce brown rice or teff flour

salt and pepper to taste

In a large saucepan add extra virgin olive oil and on medium-low heat add sliced onions; fry for a few minutes. Wash tomatoes, and cook under low heat with the onions for 10 minutes, with the pan covered. Then, add water and allspice; stew gently for about a half hour. String through sieve and return to saucepan. Work butter and flour into a ball, and place in the soup. Boil gently until dissolved. Add dried basil and oregano and serve.

Puree of Spinach Soup (thyroid, pituitary)

2 pounds organic spinach, well washed

1½ pints vegetable stock

½ pint hot organic whole milk

1 ounce brown rice flour

1 ounce organic butter

1 teaspoon minced onion

1 yolk organic egg or 2 T. organic cream

½ teaspoon Red Sour Grape Powder (optional)

sprinkle or two of nutmeg

small amount freshly ground black pepper

sea salt to taste

Clean wilted spinach and remove stocks. Wash thoroughly. Once washed, put dripping wet into a saucepan with a half teaspoonful of salt; cover the pan and let contents boil gently until soft. Drain off all fluid to eliminate potassium, and add a bit more water; reheat until hot, and discard this water. Melt butter in another pan, and stir flour smoothly into it; add stock, and stir over heat until boiling. Drain, press, and add spinach, also the onion, and re-boil for 5 minutes. Rub the soup through a fine sieve and add enough hot milk to make it as thick as heavy cream, and heat nearly to boiling. Then, add beaten yolk of egg or cream and season carefully. Serve immediately.

Simple Avocado and Tomato Salad (all types)

2 large avocados, skin removed, halved, and seeded

3 large tomatoes
1 medium red onion, peeled
Uncorrupted Balsamic Vinegar
extra virgin olive oil or crude, cold-pressed, fortified pumpkinseed oil
sea salt

Cut avocados into slices. Cut tomatoes into wedges (about six per tomato). Slice the onion. Place alternating wedges of tomato and avocado on a platter and top with onion; drizzle with oil and vinegar and add sea salt, as desired.

Romaine and Feta Cheese Salad (all types)

2 cups romaine lettuce, chopped
1 medium carrot, sliced
½ organic red sweet pepper, chopped
2 red radishes, sliced
3 T. crumbled feta cheese
extra virgin olive oil or Poppy Seed Oil
Elderberry or Grape Balsamic Vinegar (high quality, no sulfites or caramel)

Mix all salad ingredients and top with oil and vinegar.

Cucumber Pickled Salad (thyroid, muscular, pituitary)

3 cucumbers with tender skins
3 Wild Cucumbers (Asmar's Pickled Brand, optional)
½ yellow onion, diced
a few cherry tomatoes
Gegenbauer Raw Cucumber Vinegar
extra virgin olive oil
sea salt

Slice cucumbers and remove skin, if tough. If no wild cucumbers are available, use organic dill pickles. Mix all salad ingredients and top with desired amount of Cucumber Vinegar, extra virgin olive oil, and salt

Simple Yogurt-Cucumber Salad (all types)

2 medium cucumbers, peeled, sliced, and quartered
2 or more cups full fat yogurt
a bit of dried or fresh mint
sea salt to taste

In yogurt add cucumbers and salt; sprinkle or top with mint.

Endocrine note: This may also be consumed for adrenal types by adding extra salt. The yogurt helps neutralize any overpowering effect of excess potassium on the adrenal glands.

Metabolic Salad (thyroid, muscular, and pituitary)

1 cup organic dandelion greens
1 cup organic romaine lettuce
¼ cup organic purslane
2 T. fresh organic parsley, chopped
3 or 4 wedges organic avocado
a few pine nuts
3 T. rare remote-source vinegar such as Black Currant or Honey Vinegar
    (if unavailable, use organic apple cider vinegar)
3 T. extra virgin olive oil or Crude Cold-Pressed Pumpkinseed Oil
1-2 teaspoons Wild Super-5-Greens Juice (optional)

Mix all salad ingredients; lay avocado over the top and top with a few pine nuts. Pour over vinegar, Super-Greens, and oil.

Endocrine note: This salad is ideal for pituitary types. This is particularly true of people with the anterior pituitary type, who are bloated or pear shaped. The dandelion greens, purslane, and Super-Greens Juice help cleanse any congestion from the liver as well as the kidneys.

Salmon and Chopped Vegetable Salad (all types, especially pituitary and thyroid)

1 large can wild salmon, drained

2 stalks celery, chopped

2 parsley roots, sliced and quartered

1 medium onion, chopped

2 medium carrots, sliced and quartered

8 red radishes, chopped

extra virgin olive oil or Poppy Seed Oil

a good Uncontaminated Balsamic Vinegar (Seggiano is ideal)

sea salt to taste

1 teaspoon Super-5-Greens Juice (optional)

In a medium bowl add salmon plus a fourth of the juice. Add chopped vegetables and vinegar plus wild greens juice; mix until well blended. Serve by scooping on platter. Quantity of oil and vinegar depends upon consistency desired.

Endocrine note: The wild greens juice helps flush any mercury from the body. This helps prevent mercury toxicity to the endocrine glands.

Simple Sardine Salad (thyroid, pituitary)

1 can sardines in water

2 cups chopped organic lettuce

1 medium tomato, diced

1 medium yellow onion, diced

some crumbled wild oregano

juice of half lemon

Mix salad greens, tomato, and onion; layer with sardines and top with lemon juice and oregano.

Cherry Tomato Salad (all types)

20 organic cherry tomatoes, halved

1 medium red onion, diced

2 T. parsley, chopped

1 medium organic cucumber, diced

extra virgin olive oil and balsamic vinegar, as desired

chunks of organic feta or Monterey Jack cheese

plenty of sea salt to taste

Add all ingredients, and pour on desired amount of extra virgin olive oil and vinegar. Adrenal types should always add either feta cheese or Monterey Jack cheese. Salt liberally.

Endocrine note: Remember, the salt is needed to help maintain blood volume. People with this type lack the hormone necessary to cause salt and water retention. Thus, the added salt is crucial for maintaining mere normal physiology. The potassium in vegetables antagonizes this. So, this is why the salt must be added.

Chopped Root Salad (adrenal, muscular)

2 turnips, chopped

2 parsnips, chopped

2 parsley roots, chopped

1/2 C raw, pickled turnip (optional)

1 raw potato, chopped (optional)

1 small onion, chopped

bits of cheese

Mix all ingredients. Top with crude cold-pressed pumpkinseed oil, cold-pressed sesame oil, or extra virgin olive oil. Ideal vinegars are balsamic, Red Sweet Pepper, and Elderberry Balsamic.

Beefsteak Tomato with Feta Salad (all types)

2 huge tomatoes
1 large red onion
a few fresh basil leaves
crumbled feta cheese
a few pine nuts, raw or toasted

Slice tomatoes thick. Slice onion medium-thick. Interface tomato and onion; top with remaining ingredients. Drizzle with balsamic vinegar and extra virgin olive oil, if desired.

Vegetable Cottage Cheese Salad (adrenal, muscular, thyroid)

2 parsnips, chopped
1 large organic red sweet pepper, diced
2 cups organic full fat cottage cheese

Mix all ingredients and serve as a side dish. Or, eat as an entire meal.

Hot Cottage Cheese Salad (adrenal, muscular)

4 red or white radishes, chopped
1 medium red onion, diced
1 medium turnip, diced
2 cups organic full fat cottage cheese
small amount freshly grated horseradish (or horseradish sauce)

Mix all ingredients, and serve chilled on a platter with an ice cream scoop.

Chopped Tomato, Onion, and Cucumber Salad with Balsamic/Pomegranate Dressing (all types)

2 whole medium organic cucumbers

4 whole medium to large organic tomatoes

2 medium red onions

wild oregano from either wild bunches or Crude Wild Oregano Capsules

sea salt to taste

For dressing:

4 T. High Quality Uncolored and Uncorrupted Balsamic Vinegar (Seggiano is ideal)

1 T. Pom-o-Power Mediterranean Sour Pomegranate Syrup

4 T. extra virgin olive oil or Crude Cold-Pressed Pumpkinseed Oil

Dice all vegetables and toss with crushed fresh or dried wild oregano. Mix dressing and pour as desired.

Endocrine note: In particular, thyroid types benefit from pomegranate concentrate, since they are vulnerable to circulatory disorders and such a concentrate is protective against this. Also, adrenal types can also use this recipe by aggressively salting the vegetables/salad.

Vegetable and Side Dishes

Fried Artichokes (all types)

1 pound artichokes, cut in spears

1 raw whole organic egg

2 T. brown rice flour

teaspoon Red Sour Grape Powder

sea salt

teaspoon lemon juice
Village-Made Wild Red Palm Oil

Brush artichokes with egg, dust with brown rice flour and red sour grape; leave until dry. Then, repeat the process. In a saucepan heat Red Palm Oil and fry artichokes; drain well, sprinkle with salt and lemon juice and serve. For adrenal types be sure to salt the artichokes well.

Fried Artichokes Au Parmesan (all types)

1 pound artichokes
2 ounces grated full fat organic cheese
Wild Village-Made Red Palm Oil (or use organic butter)
small amount of brown rice flour
a little whole organic milk

Wash and peel artichokes, and either steam them over fast-boiling water or if late in the season, boil them in milk and water to keep them white. Drain well, and brush with egg and roll in brown rice flour. Fry in Red Palm Oil and sprinkle with cheese.

Endocrine note: artichokes are a good food for the pancreas. They also help balance liver function. These wonder-vegetables help adrenal function by balancing blood sugar levels.

Fried Cucumber (all types)

2 organic cucumbers
3 T. brown rice flour
Wild Village-Made Red Palm Oil or organic butter (large amount is needed)

Cut cucumbers into pieces about 1½ inches long and peel them. Dry carefully in a cloth; put flour in a bag and toss until coated. Have pan ready with oil (or butter) and heat on medium heat. Fry cucumbers carefully until flour layer is brown and serve hot. Salt liberally.

Endocrine note: frying vegetables makes them more suitable for adrenal types; also, the fat is used by the body as energy, which is needed in all types. This is why this is a universal recipe.

Baked Tomatoes with Oregano and Garlic (all types; for adrenals salt heavily)

6 organic plum tomatoes, cut in half

4 T. extra virgin olive oil

1 clove garlic, minced

high quality Wild Oregano from Bunches or contents three Crude Wild
    Oregano/Rhus Capsules

2 T. chopped fresh parsley

1 T. chopped fresh basil (optional)

½ oz. Organic Rice Bran

sea salt and freshly ground black pepper

In a large frying pan heat oil. Add tomatoes, cut-side down and cook over low heat for about six minutes, turning over after four minutes.

In an oven-safe dish place cooked tomatoes and sprinkle with salt and pepper to taste, garlic, oregano, parsley, and basil, then rice bran. Drizzle with remaining oil from frying pan; bake in a preheated oven at 350 degrees Fahrenheit for about 40 minutes.

Escalloped Eggplant (all types)

Again, the addition of eggs, cream, or milk to vegetables makes these vegetable dishes ideal for adrenal types. This is a highly rich recipe loaded with nutrients, including the much needed cholesterol for hormone production.

2 eggplants

1 cup organic cream

2 organic egg yolks

2 T. organic butter
sea salt, wild oregano, and pepper

Beat eggs slightly. Peel and cut eggplants, and soak for an hour in salt water. Drain and cook in boiling water until tender. Drain again thoroughly and mash. Add butter, cream, and egg yolks. Beat all together well, and turn into well buttered casserole. Top with bits of butter and brown in a hot oven.

Fried Wild Rice topped with Organic Yogurt (all types)

³/₄ cup real Wild Rice, 100% northern Canadian, rinsed
sea salt or Herbamere
1 yellow onion, diced
¹/₂ organic green pepper, diced
¹/₂ cup organic yogurt
heavy fat (such as Wild Red Palm Oil, clarified butter, or extra virgin
    olive oil)
contents of 2 Crude Wild Oregano (OregaMax) capsules (optional)

In a pot add four or more cups pure water plus sea salt or Herbamere and cover. Heat until boiling; add wild rice and heat for 30 seconds; turn off heat and keep covered (this will prevent excessive cooking; the hot water will cook it).

In a frying pan heat oil and add onion and green pepper. Cook for five minutes, and add rice and seasoning. Cook until rice is completely hot. Serve with a dollop of full fat yogurt: a complete meal.

Stewed Mushrooms (mainly thyroid, muscular, adrenal)

Mushrooms are high in selenium, a mineral desperately needed by the thyroid gland. Parsnips contain special substances that are anti-tumor.

¹/₂ pound organic mushrooms of any kind

1 pint organic whole milk

1 ounce organic butter (or Wild Village-Made Red Palm Oil)

1 or 2 ounces brown rice flour

green stems of two green onions

sea salt and lemon juice

Peel and stalk mushrooms, wash them quickly but carefully. Put in a saucepan with milk, and let them cook gently until they are tender. Mix the flour smoothly and thinly with a little cold milk, then add this to the mushrooms and milk mixture; stir over the heat until it boils well and thickens. Season to taste and garnish with small slices of green onion.

Spaghetti Squash Vegetarian Spaghetti (all types, especially pituitary)

1 spaghetti squash, outside well cleaned

1 jar Antica Italia Puttanesca (special imported Italian pasta sauce)

4 T. pine nuts

1 red onion, chopped

2 T. English walnuts, chunked

2 cloves garlic, chopped

extra virgin olive oil

Bake spaghetti squash. In a large frying pan heat a few tablespoons extra virgin olive oil; add pine nuts, walnuts, garlic, and onions; cook until browned. When spaghetti squash is done, add about 3/4 of the jar of Puttanesca sauce to the frying pan; cook until hot and well blended. With a fork pull out spaghetti squash, and place evenly on plates. Pour on sauce and serve—a delicious and healthy treat.

Red Potato and Onion Stew, Indian-Style (adrenal, muscular)

2 lb. organic red potatoes, washed, diced

bunch organic spring onions, skin removed, chopped

1 teaspoon fenugreek seeds
1 teaspoon shredded ginger
1 teaspoon curry powder
½ teaspoon freshly ground pepper
1 cup organic vegetable stock
Poppy Seed Oil or extra virgin olive oil
sea salt

Brown fenugreek seeds in oil for one minute. Then, add ginger for another minute or so. Sprinkle curry powder over mixture. Add diced potatoes and chopped onions. Season with salt and pepper; pour in stock. Cook over low heat until potatoes are done and stock is nearly gone.

Parsnip Croquettes (mainly muscular and pituitary)

6 large parsnips
2 whole organic eggs
large amount butter or Wild Village-Made Red Palm Oil
a small amount of whole wheat flour
teaspoon Red Sour Grape Powder (Resvital, optional)
sea salt and pepper
rice bran crumbs

Wash and scrub parsnips, then boil until tender. Drain off water, and let them get cold. Next, peel them, and either rub them through a sieve or grate them. Beat two eggs, and add to parsnip, mixing thoroughly. Then, sprinkle in enough flour to bind mixture. Mix in red sour grape (if possible) and spread evenly on a plate; make it in even divisions, flour the hands slightly, and shape into small balls. Brush each ball with beaten egg on all sides, then cover with rice bran crumbs. In a saucepan heat butter or Wild Red Palm Oil; use enough fat to nearly cover balls. Fry until golden yellow. Place on brown paper towels to drain, and serve immediately.

Entrees

Brown Lentil Stew (mainly adrenal and muscular)

½ pound brown lentils

1 pint water

1 pound organic tomatoes

1 pound yellow onions

2 ounces organic butter

¼ teaspoon Marmite (yeast extract)

sea salt and pepper

Wash lentils. In a pan boil water. Add lentils and simmer gently for 3 hours. Slice and fry onions in butter (or use wild-source red palm oil) until nicely brown. Peel tomatoes and add to onions, and cook for ½ hour. Then, add the cooked lentils, and stew all together for another ½ hour. Season, and add Marmite just before serving dissolved in a small amount of water. If the stew is too thin add brown rice or whole wheat flour to thicken. Serve with steamed cabbage. Salt the cabbage liberally, and put Parsley Butter on it.

Organic Cheese Omelet (thyroid, adrenal, muscular)

3 large organic eggs

1 large tablespoonful grated organic Monterey Jack or cheddar cheese

1 ounce butter or 2 T. Wild Village-Made Red Palm Oil

1 T. whole organic milk

sea salt

Break eggs into a bowl, and beat to a light froth; add milk and three-parts cheese. Season with pepper and salt. Melt butter in omelet-pan; pour in egg mixture. Stir gently over a medium heat until eggs are about half set; then, tip the pan wells up and roll mixture over until it forms an oval cushion. Turn the omelet on to a hot dish, and sprinkle surface with remaining cheese and serve immediately.

Note: there is no calcium in eggs. By adding milk and cheese this fortifies the nutrition of the eggs, making a highly nutritionally dense meal. This is why it is ideal for thyroid, thyroid-muscular, and adrenal types.

Feta Cheese Mediterranean Omelet (mainly adrenal, thyroid, and muscular)

3 large organic eggs

2 T. organic feta cheese

1 T. chopped parsley

3 T. extra virgin olive oil

1 T. whole organic milk

1/2 teaspoon oregano from Wild Oregano Bunches

sea salt to taste

Crack eggs and whip well, adding milk. In a skillet heat extra virgin olive oil; add eggs and cook until half set. Sprinkle feta cheese and oregano and tilt pan and flip (or turn with a large spoon/spatula). When nearly done sprinkle with parsley and serve hot.

Alpine Eggs (all types but mainly adrenal and thyroid)

4 organic eggs

4 ounces grated organic Monterey Jack or other white cheese

1 1/2 ounces organic butter

1 small onion

1/2 teaspoon chopped parsley

small amount wild oregano

sea salt and pepper

Mince onion and fry in butter, until light brown. Pour into fire-proof baking dish. Sprinkle thickly with cheese. Carefully break eggs over cheese, dust with pepper and a bit of oregano (if desired), cover with grated cheese, with small bits of butter on top. Bake in a pre-heated oven (450 degrees or more) for about 10 minutes and serve immediately.

Savory Organic Eggs (all types, but mainly adrenal and thyroid)

6 hard-boiled organic eggs

2 T. curry paste

2 ounces organic butter

2 T. tomato juice

Shell eggs, and cut in half around the egg (the short way). Remove yolks, being careful not to break whites. Put yolks in a bowl with butter, and work both together with a wooden spoon; then, add the curry and tomato juice. Season the mixture with a bit of salt and pepper, if desired. Then, rub it through a sieve or gravy strainer. Fill the empty egg whites with egg yolk mixture and chill. Serve arranged on a bed of salad greens.

Lamb (or beef) Kidneys with Raisins and Thyme (all types)

8 organic kidneys

4 T. organic butter (or 4 T. wild Village-Made Red Palm Oil)

1 medium red onion, sliced

3 sprigs thyme

a few cloves

4 ounces raisin juice (or in 3 oz. water add 2 T. Grape Molasses)

handful raisins

In a saucepan heat butter; cook onion until brown. Cut kidneys in half, rinse, and pat dry. Reheat pan and add, cooking on low heat and covered for about 10 minutes, turning several times. Heat raisin juice, cloves, and thyme in separate pot and cook nearly until boiling. Add raisins and pour over kidneys. Cook on minimal heat for 5 or 6 minutes.

Chicken Marguerite (mainly adrenal but also thyroid)

2 young or small organic chickens
1 pint organic cream
a few sultanas (optional)
sea salt, pepper, and paprika

Cut chicken, like a frying chicken; be sure to remove the wings from the breast pieces. Sauté in butter until well done and browned. Pour cream and sultanas into the pan just before the chicken is done. Season and serve.

Braised Organic Chicken with Thyme (adrenal, thyroid)

4½ pounds organic chicken pieces, cleaned and dried
2 T. organic butter
2 T. Wild Village-Made Red Palm Oil (if unavailable, use extra butter)
1 cup organic tomatoes
4 large organic carrots, sliced
1 onion, sliced
¼ teaspoon paprika
parsley
thyme
bay leaf
sea salt and pepper

On medium heat melt butter in large frying pan; lay in chicken, turning on all sides until brown. Remove from frying pan and place in large casserole. Pour over butter and add all other ingredients; add boiling water to half the height of the meat. Cover tightly and bake in oven at low heat until tender. Baste often and add more water, if necessary. Serve with carrots and onions around chicken. Strain liquid and make into gravy, if desired.

Sardines au Gratin (mainly pituitary)

6 ripe tomatoes

chopped parsley

2 tins boneless skinless sardines

½ cup grated organic Parmesan cheese

5 teaspoons organic chicken stock

organic butter

garlic

sea salt

Peel tomatoes and remove seeds. In a pan stew in butter with garlic, parsley, and salt, along with chicken stock. Put a layer of the tomatoes on the bottom of a shallow gratin dish. Place the sardines on top and cover with another layer of tomatoes. Sprinkle with grated Parmesan cheese and brown in oven.

Simple Grilled Fish (all types)

your selection of one pound fish fillets, any type

extra virgin olive oil or Natural Remote-Source Poppy Seed Oil, plus
    Uncorrupted Balsamic Vinegar (for marinade)

garlic salt

onion salt

Marinate fish in oil and vinegar and dust with garlic/onion salt. Grill to desired doneness, being careful not to over-cook. Serve Hawaiian-style with slices of papaya (aids in digestion).

Organic Pot Roast (adrenal, thyroid, muscular)

1 piece bottom round of organic beef

5 fresh tomatoes

2 cloves

8 small organic carrots

Village-Made Wild Palm Oil or organic butter, as needed

vegetable stock, as needed

2 bay leaves, a few sprigs of thyme, and parsley tied together

8 small onions

2 medium parsnips, peeled and quartered

In a large pan brown beef in butter on all sides (or use Wild Red Palm Oil). Remove and set in casserole. Fry onions and carrots in same butter (or Red Palm Oil) and put in casserole. Add remaining ingredients and enough vegetable stock to cover them. Bring to a boil on top of stove; cover tightly and place in moderate oven for two hours. Remove meat from casserole. Strain sauce through colander. Serve with vegetables surrounding meat and sauce poured over them.

Note: the meat juices are full of nutrients, plus much needed fats from the meats. The fats include cholesterol needed by the adrenal glands, ovaries, and testes. For people with adrenal types, including thyroid-adrenal, this is an ideal recipe.

Simple Steak 'n Onions (mainly adrenal, muscular, and thyroid)

2 organic steaks, any type

1 large red onion

a bit of sumac (if available) or contents of two wild oregano complex capsules.

Slice onions. In a skillet cook onions and steaks to desired doneness, although the meat is healthiest in medium- to medium-rare; sprinkle with sumac.

Simple Sweet Thai Shrimp Curry (mainly adrenal and pituitary)

1 14 fl. oz (400 ml) can coconut milk

3 cups (or a bit more) pure water

3 T. Thai red curry paste or to taste

½ lb. wild shrimp (or prawns cut in chunks), cleaned and deveined

1 T. dried lemongrass (or a whole lemongrass stalk, chopped)

about 1 inch fresh ginger root

1 T. raw honey

juice of one or two limes

2 oz. button mushrooms, sliced

fresh cilantro leaves

Heat water and coconut milk to a boil. Crush lemongrass with the flat of a chef's knife once, then cut into ½-inch chunks. Slice ginger root into thin rounds. Reserve these, along with lime juice. When soup base has boiled, add these ingredients. Add honey, curry paste, and boil for 2 or 3 minutes. Add shrimps, mushrooms, and lime juice; lower to medium-high heat. Cook for only 2 or 3 minutes, until the shrimps have turned white and springy; do not overcook. Transfer to soup tureen and serve garnished with cilantro leaves.

Incredible Creamy Chicken Curry (thyroid, muscular, adrenal)

4 organic chicken breasts, skin on

1 cup organic chicken or turkey stock

3 yellow onions, diced

2 cloves garlic, diced

1 teaspoon fresh ginger, grated

2 organic tomatoes, peeled and chopped

1 red or green pepper, cored and finely chopped

½ teaspoon freshly ground cumin seed

½ teaspoon freshly ground coriander seed

¼ teaspoon curry powder

Wild Red Palm Oil (Village-Made)

Real Hand-picked Native Wild Rice, cooked

sea salt, as needed

Cut chicken into small pieces and set aside. In a saucepan brown onion in Red Palm Oil. Add chicken, garlic, and ginger; brown over medium heat for about 3 minutes. Add tomatoes, finely chopped pepper, and cup of chicken stock. Stir and simmer over medium heat for about 5 minutes. Add spices and stir again. Check salt and add more, if needed, and on a high heat cook until the liquids have reduced to a thickness. Serve hot over a bed of Real Hand-Picked Wild Rice, the latter being a super-rich source of B vitamins.

Lamb Chops, Greek Style (all types, but mainly thyroid and adrenal)

four organic lamb chops
half lemon
dried oregano from Wild Oregano Bunches
teaspoon Red Sour Grape Powder (optional but tasty and nutritious)

In a skillet over medium low heat cook lamb chops, retaining all fat. Sprinkle with spices and squeeze lemon. If desired, add sliced onions. Serve and pour any remaining grease over the finished meat. Note: grilled lamb is exceptionally nourishing for people with adrenal body types.

Baked Whole Fish, Middle Eastern-Style (all types)

one whole fish of any kind
2 T. extra virgin olive oil
½ cup pine nuts
1 large red onion, finely chopped
¼ cup currants or golden raisins

Clean whole fish. Mix all ingredients and stuff in center. Bake at 300°until done.

Really Good Indian Lamb Stew (all types, especially adrenal)

1 pound organic lamb, cubed

1 large onion, diced

2 cloves garlic, diced

1 teaspoon ginger, finely chopped

2 ripe organic tomatoes, chopped

3 pints organic full fat yogurt

1 T. pine nuts

1 green (or red) pepper, cored, de-seeded, and chopped

2 bay leaves

1 teaspoon freshly ground coriander

Cold-Pressed Poppy Seed Oil or Sesame Oil

sea salt

raw honey

a few pomegranate seeds

Heat about 3 tablespoons oil in a skillet; cook onions, garlic, tomatoes, peppers, ginger, bay leaf, coriander, pine nuts, and lamb; add a pinch of sea salt. Add a half teaspoon raw honey. Fry for a few minutes until lamb is partially browned. Then add yogurt, and simmer over very low heat for about 26 minutes. Stir every few minutes. Serve hot. Garnish with a few pomegranate seeds and chopped coriander.

Organic Chicken Breast ala Pomegranate (all types)

4 T. extra virgin olive oil (Estate-Made, such as Seggiano)

2 red onions, thinly sliced

$\frac{1}{2}$ teaspoon turmeric

3 cups walnuts

4 cups organic chicken stock

4 organic chicken breasts, skin on

2 pomegranates

3 T. Mediterranean Pomegranate Extract, Sour Type (Pom-o-Power)

3 T. lemon juice

1 or 2 teaspoons Red Sour Grape Powder (optional)

1 T. raw honey (optional)

sea salt

wild oregano from bunches (or use contents of OregaMax capsules)

In a skillet heat onions and add turmeric. Cook until limp. Transfer to a saucepan, adding organic chicken stock, walnuts, and seasoning. Stir and bring to a boil. Uncovered, simmer for about 20 minutes.

Cut in half pomegranates and seed. Reserve the seeds. In a skillet add 2 T. olive oil; add chicken breasts and cook until done, turning when needed. Transfer to a prewarmed plate until needed. To the same pan add pomegranate extract (Pom-o-Power), plus lemon juice and red sour grape (optional); stir with wooden spoon, adding the stock/walnut/onion mixture; simmer until the sauce thickens slightly. Serve chicken breasts sliced, drizzled with sauce and pomegranate seeds. Excess sauce can be put in a sauce bowl.

Yogurt with Cucumbers and Mint (all types; beware, some people with pituitary types have mint allergies)

1 whole cucumber, peeled

3 T. finely chopped mint

a few sprigs, as garnish

1 or 2 cloves garlic, crushed

1 teaspoon raw honey

1½ cup organic whole fat yogurt

1 teaspoon sea salt

Slice cucumber into spears, then chop. Combine chopped cucumber with sea salt; leave for 20 minutes. Salt softens cucumbers. Combine mint, garlic, and honey, along with yogurt, in bowl. Rinse cucumber in sieve to remove salt. Drain well and add to yogurt mixture. Garnish with a few sprigs of mint.

Special Sauteed Organic Calves' or Lamb's Liver (all types, especially pituitary)

1 pound organic liver
crushed wild oregano from either Capsules of Wild Oregano or freshly
    ground oregano leaves (from bunches)
Red Sour Grape
garlic salt
onion salt
1 medium onion, sliced
extra virgin olive oil or Wild Village-Made Red Palm Oil

Rinse and slice liver; pat dry. In a plastic bag add sufficient amount of
the spices/seasonings. Add liver, a piece at a time, and coat. In a large
skillet heat oil; add slices of liver, along with onion, and cook on low
heat for a few minutes; avoid over-cooking, as liver should be pinkish
red in the center when serving.

Grilled Sour Prawns (all types)

8 prawns
2 T. extra virgin olive oil or Seggiano Lemon-Flavored Olive Oil
juice of two lemons
teaspoon Red Sour Grape Powder
2 teaspoons diced fresh cilantro

Marinate prawns in all the above ingredients. Grill until done and serve
    hot.

Baked Halibut (all types)

2 halibut fillets
1 medium red onion
lemon wedges

small amount chopped fresh parsley
1 teaspoon red sour grape powder (optional)

Wash fillets and place on a baking pan. Slice onion and place slices on fish; sprinkle on red sour grape powder. Pre-heat oven to 250 degrees. Cook until just hot in the center (do not over-cook or fish will become dry). Serve and squeeze lemon wedges, and top with chopped parsley.

Endocrine note: while mercury is a problem halibut is an excellent source of vitamins and minerals as well as a top source of protein and omega 3 fish oils. In particular, it is an ideal food for pituitary and adrenal types. The red sour grape powder (blue label brand) helps naturally lower cholesterol, plus it helps purge from the body noxious heavy metals such as mercury.

Grilled Marinated Wild Salmon with Pine Nuts (all types)

2 wild salmon fillets
Marinade:
2 or 3 T. extra virgin olive oil
2 T. fine Uncorrupted Balsamic Vinegar or Raw Pure Honey Vinegar
a few pine nuts, well crushed
clove of garlic, crushed
teaspoon Red Sour Grape Powder (if available)
a few extra pine nuts
a few cherry tomatoes
1 or 2 teaspoons Super-5-Greens Juice (optional)

In a ceramic container add all ingredients for marinade and add salmon. Cover and let soak for a few hours or preferably overnight. Grill salmon and cherry tomatoes, being sure not to over-cook. Simultaneously, in a small skillet toast pine nuts in olive oil. When salmon is done, place on a hot plate and surround with a few cherry tomatoes, topping with pine nuts.

Endocrine note: be sure the salmon is wild. Farm raised salmon is poisonous and will disrupt endocrine function. This type of salmon contains up to 16 times more PCBs and other pollutants than the wild type. For truly wild and remote-source salmon see Americanwildfoods.com.

Fried Organic or Grass-Fed Minute Steak (ideal for adrenal, also thyroid and muscular)

4 organic minute steaks
2 T. organic butter or Village-Made Red Palm Oil

In a heavy skillet add Red Palm Oil or butter until quite hot. Sear steaks quickly on both sides, lower heat, and cook for about 2 minutes on each side. Remove and add salt; serve immediately. Optional: dust steaks in a high quality whole grain flour before cooking.

Tasty Marinated Lamb Chops (thyroid, adrenal, muscular)

4 or more organic lamb chops
Marinade:
3 T. Poppy Seed Oil or extra virgin olive oil
2 T. Raw Quince Vinegar or Uncorrupted Balsamic Vinegar
a pinch of Pure Rosemary Spice (ground into a powder)
1 bay leaf
clove garlic, crushed
a few clumps of wild oregano (from Wild Oregano Crunches)
a few basil leaves
1 T. Sour Pomegranate Molasses (blue label brand)

In a deep ceramic dish place lamb chops; in a separate bowl add all marinade ingredients and mix; then, pour over lamb chops. Allow to marinate for at least 4 hours and preferably overnight. In a skillet cook lamb chops over medium-low heat; baste with marinade and serve.

Vitamin-Burger (thyroid, adrenal, muscular)

1 pound ground grass-fed or organic beef
3 T. Organic non-GMO Rice Bran
1 T. wheat germ (optional)
1 teaspoon Herbamere
½ teaspoon onion salt
½ teaspoon garlic salt
thick onion slices for grilling, if desired

In a bowl thoroughly mix all ingredients. Make into hamburgers of desired thickness and cook. Serve hot with exotic Cranberry Ketchup and Cuban Mustard. Eat on a platter, without a bun.

Low-Carb Vitamin-Rich Beef Stew (muscular and adrenal)

2 pounds lean organic beef cut into 1-inch cubes
3 T. organic butter or Village-Made Red Palm Oil
1 large onion, chopped
4 medium turnips, cut into bite-sized chunks
3 medium spears broccoli, cut into chunks
12 Brussels sprouts, well washed, outer spoiled leaves removed
2 parsley roots, sliced (optional but tasty)
8 small white onions
2 T. Organic non-GMO Rice Bran or brown rice flour
2 teaspoons Red Sour Grape Powder (optional)
organic beef broth, heated

In a large heavy skillet melt butter or Red Palm Oil. Sprinkle in meat and brown, then adding chopped onion. Add the heated broth, enough to nearly cover the meat. Cover, and simmer slowly for 2 hours over low heat (or until nearly done). Then add whole onions, Brussels sprouts, broccoli, turnips, and parsley root. Continue simmering for another half hour. To a platter remove meat and vegetables. Thicken the remaining liquid in a large pot, along with the rice bran or flour until mixed to a smooth paste. Use this as a gravy for the stew.

Vitamin Liver (all types, especially thyroid)

1 pound fresh organic calves' or lamb's liver,
1 or 2 T. organic butter or Village-Made Red Palm Oil
1 large yellow onion, sliced
3 or more T. Organic (non-GMO) Rice Bran
3 green onions, diced
sea salt

Rinse liver, slice, and pat dry. In a plastic bag add bran; add liver, a piece at a time, and coat lightly. In a heavy skillet heat butter or oil and add the yellow onion, placing the onion on the sides. After cooking for 2 or 3 minutes add the liver sprinkled with green onions, and cook no more than an additional 3 minutes. Sprinkle with sea salt and serve.

Endocrine note: this is a truly B vitamin-rich meal, since both liver and rice bran are top sources. The thyroid gland desperately needs these vitamins, as do all endocrine glands. Yet, this recipe is particularly valuable for thyroid types.

Diced Spicy Organic Liver with Onions

1 pound fresh organic beef or calves' liver sliced into cubes
2 or more T. organic butter or extra virgin olive oil
1 large yellow onion, diced
2 T. bulk wild oregano/Rhus coriaria complex
1 T. powdered Red Sour Grape
1 teaspoon ground coriander or curry powder
1/2 teaspoon sea salt

Wash liver and drain. Pat dry. Place half liver in Ziploc bag, and add half the spices. Shake until well coated. Repeat for the remainder of the liver. In a skillet on medium-low heat butter or oil. Add onions, and cook for two minutes. Add liver, and cook for five minutes. Do not overcook.

Juicy Ribeye Steaks with Garlic and Onion (thyroid and adrenal)

2 juicy organic ribeye steaks
2 large yellow onions, cut into rings
3 cloves garlic, sliced
Wild Red Palm Oil (optional)

Wash steaks and pat dry. In a saucepan under medium-low heat (add oil and) cook steaks; add onions and garlic and allow to cook in the juices. Ideally, serve medium-rare to medium, so as to retain the juices. Top with Parsley Butter.

Spinach, Onion, and Lemon Soup with Curried Lamb Balls (thyroid and adrenal, also muscular)

2 large yellow onions
2 or 3 T. extra virgin olive oil
1 T. curry powder
½ cup garbanzo beans
2 cups minced organic lamb (use organic beef, if unavailable)
1 lb. organic spinach leaves, chopped
½ cup organic brown rice flour
juice of two lemons (or limes)
3 extra large organic eggs, beaten
2 garlic cloves, finely minced
2 tablespoons organic parsley, finely minced
sea salt and pepper to taste

Finely chop onions, and set half aside. Heat olive oil over medium heat in a large frying pan; fry onion until limp. Add curry powder, chick peas, and about 2 pints of water (or more, as needed); bring to a boil. Reduce heat and simmer for 15 to 20 minutes.

In a large mixing bowl add remaining onion, along with lamb and small amount of pepper; add a few pinches of curry. Using hands mix and form into small balls. Gently lay in saucepan and simmer for 10 minutes. Then, add spinach, cover and simmer for an additional 18 minutes.

Mix flour with 8 oz. cold water to make a smooth paste. Slowly add it to the saucepan, stirring continuously to prevent clumping. Stir in lemon juice, and season with salt and pepper. Cook for about 20 minutes (over minimal heat). Now, fry garlic in a bit of olive oil until golden. Add parsley but only cook for another minute.

Remove soup from heat and stir in eggs. Sprinkle the garlic-parsley garnish over the soup and serve.

Easy-to-Make Grape Leaf Rolls (all types)

Grape leaves are great for circulation. People with thyroid types need help in this realm. Moreover, the muscular types are vulnerable to heart disease.

2 T. extra virgin olive oil

1 cup organic minced lamb or beef

3 T. pine nuts

1 T. walnut

1 medium to large onion, chopped

1 T. tomato puree

1 T. chopped fresh coriander

1 tsp. ground cumin

$\frac{1}{2}$ tsp. mint (optional)

10 grape leaves

sea salt and pepper

⅔ cup organic beef stock

In a saucepan heat one tablespoon oil. Add meat, nuts, and onion. Cook until brown. Stir in fresh coriander, cumin, tomato puree, and mint. Cook for an additional 3 minutes, and season with salt and pepper. Preheat oven to 350 degrees Fahrenheit. Prepare a baking/casserole dish with one or more tablespoons olive oil rubbed or poured on the flat surface. Place vine leaves on a flat surface, shiny side down, and fill in the center of each leaf, then fold the stalk over the filling. Roll it towards the tip of the leaf and put in a baking/casserole dish, seam side down. Pour in beef stock. Cook covered in oven for about 30 minutes.

Paprika Chicken (adrenal and thyroid)

⅓ cup finely ground oat and rice bran flour

1 teaspoon sea salt

sprinkle or two freshly ground pepper

one 2½ to 3 pound (cut up) organic chicken

⅓ cup pure organic butter

½ cup red onion, chopped

¼ cup water

2 tablespoons Hungarian paprika

Combine flour, salt, and pepper. Coat chicken pieces with mixture. Brown chicken in butter (if allergic to butter use coconut oil) Add onion, water, and 1 tablespoon paprika. Cover; simmer for about 45 minutes. Remove pieces and keep hot. Serve with Sour Cream Gravy.

Recipe for gravy: In a pan blend 1 tablespoon oat/rice bran flour plus ¼ teaspoon salt into pan drippings, along with the remaining paprika. Add

½ cup whole milk plus ½ cup sour cream, stirring constantly until thickened and fully heated. Drizzle as desired over chicken pieces.

Bran-Coated Roasted Chicken (all types)

1 organic egg, slightly beaten
2 tablespoons water
one 2½-to 3-pound organic chicken (already cut up)
¾ cup combination oat and rice bran, finely milled
¼ cup organic butter
unbleached sea salt and freshly ground pepper
garlic salt (optional)

Mix egg, water, seasonings, and salt. Dip chicken in mixture; roll in bran. Sprinkle with salt and pepper. In a baking pan melt butter; place in chicken, and bake for about an hour at 375 degrees (or until done).

Spaghetti Squash Spaghetti (thyroid, muscular)

1 large spaghetti squash
1 pound organic ground beef
1 large onion, diced
2 cloves garlic, diced
some fresh oregano from bunches (Wild Oregano Crunches)
1 jar Anta Italia Puttanesca Pasta Sauce
freshly ground Parmesan cheese

Cook spaghetti squash until done. In the meantime in a large skillet brown meat, garlic, and onion; add oregano and simmer for a few minutes. Add sauce and cook until well mixed. On large plates using a fork pull spaghetti squash and lay on the plate evenly. Pour on sauce, as desired, and top with Parmesan cheese.

Grilled Fish Medley (all types)

This dish is basic but nourishing. Wild salmon and halibut are top sources of the much needed fatty fish oils. Shrimp offers rich amounts of iodine. The Red Sour Grape Powder adds to the sour taste, while providing valuable amounts of red grape flavonoids, tartaric acid, naturally occurring chromium, and resveratrol.

2 fillets wild salmon
2 fillets halibut
6 large shrimp
juice of one lemon or lime
Red Sour Grape Powder (optional)
extra virgin olive oil

Marinate fish overnight in lemon juice, sour grape, and extra virgin olive oil. Grill and serve hot. Dip in Peanut Sauce.

Pheasant with Apricots and Wild Rice (adrenal, muscular, pituitary)

Wild game (or farm-raised game) is the ideal food for this type. This 'lean meat' is highly nutritious, plus it is high in essential fatty acids, which aid heart and liver metabolism. One of the keys for this type is to prevent fatty accumulations in the liver. This is precisely what the essential fatty acids achieve. Wild rice is abundant in B vitamins, needed by the thyroid as well as the heart and liver. Also, use only truly wild rice from remote regions of northern Canada. Support the needs of the natives by buying their own hand-harvested material (see Americanwildfoods.com).

⅓ cup wild rice, rinsed and uncooked
2 to 3 tablespoons butter
2 fresh apricots, seeded and diced
½ teaspoon ground sage

1½ to 3 pound pheasant
teaspoon garlic powder.
sea salt

All-natural basting sauce consisting of 4 tablespoons extra virgin olive oil, a few drops of oil of wild oregano (edible type, hand-picked Mediterranean), a capsule or two of crude red grape powder, and a quarter teaspoon garlic powder.

Add water and salt to a saucepan with wild rice; cook, boiling gently until just tender. Stir in softened butter, apricots, and sage plus ¼ teaspoon sea salt. Season the inside of the pheasant with sea salt. Stuff the bird with the wild rice-apricot stuffing. Truss; then place breast side up on rack in shallow pan. Roast, uncovered, at 350 degrees until tender, about 1 to 2½ hours (time varies with size and toughness). Baste occasionally and extensively with basting sauce and also drippings. Serve and pour drippings over meat.

Endocrine note: animals love meat drippings/juice. This is because this is rich in hormones and pre-hormones, including vitamins A and D. Meat drippings with sea salt is strength-producing, especially for adrenal types.

Chopped Salmon Salad (all types)

1 large can wild salmon (retain ½ juice)

2 stalks celery, chopped

1 green pepper, cored and seeded, chopped

6 red radishes, sliced

8 cherry tomatoes, cut in half

2 dill pickles, diced

extra virgin olive oil or Poppy Seed Oil and high quality Uncontaminated
    Balsamic Vinegar

sea salt

2 teaspoons Super-5-Greens Juice

In a mixing bowl add all ingredients; add also juice from the salmon; mix well. Add oil and vinegar to desired taste and salt to taste.

Lobster in Cream Sauce (mainly adrenal and pituitary)

2 lobsters, boiled
4 T. organic butter
4 large mushrooms, sliced
2 T. chopped fresh parsley
1 cup cream sauce (made from a combination of one cup whole milk with 1 or 2 T. whole wheat or rice flour)
1 or 2 T. strong Grape Molasses from Mediterranean grapes
2 T. Parmesan cheese
paprika to taste

Stir grape molasses into ½ cup water. Cut lobsters lengthwise. Remove all meat from shell and claws and slice into pieces. Do not discard shells. Heat butter and sauté mushrooms for 4 minutes, then add lobster. Slowly add cream sauce. Add parsley and grape molasses mixture and cook for 2 minutes. Put mixture back into lobster shells, sprinkle with grated cheese, and dust with paprika. In a hot oven (400 degrees) bake for 12 minutes or until cheese is browned.

Sauces, Dressings, and Miscellaneous

Incredibly Nutritious Peanut Sauce (thyroid, adrenal, muscular)

½ to 1 cup Organic Rice Bran and brown rice flour mix
½ cup finely chopped peanuts
½ cup organic heavy cream
2 or 3 T. organic butter
Herbamere to taste

dash or two paprika

teaspoon Red Sour Grape Powder (optional)

Melt butter and set aside. Mix Organic Rice Bran/flour and chopped peanuts in a small mixing bowl with cream. Add spices to melted butter and combine to make a smooth, creamy sauce.

Organic Creamy Cheese Mayonnaise (thyroid, adrenal, muscular)

1-3 oz. package organic cream cheese

2 teaspoons lemon or lime juice

1 teaspoon onion juice

½ teaspoon mild-flavored raw honey (for instance, Italian sunflower honey, clover honey, or Canadian Wild Flower Honey)

1 teaspoon coarse sea salt

4 T. Multi-Seed Oil or Poppy Seed Oil

Add all ingredients to a blender or food processor except oil and begin blending slowly. Slowly add oil, blending slowly until a creamy mayonnaise results.

Creamy Raw Berry Dressing (all types)

handful raspberries

handful blackberries

2 teaspoons Wild Blackberry Extract, Raw

3 T. Canadian Remote-Source Wild Flower Honey, Raw

5 T. organic heavy cream

Puree berries; in a mixing bowl add berry puree, Blackberry Extract, honey, and cream, and mix until even. Serve immediately or chilled over fresh fruit.

Honey-Lime Creamy Dressing (adrenal, muscular)

2 T. wild oregano or Canadian wild flower honey
5 T. organic heavy cream
5 T. lime juice
pinch or two sea salt

Mix all ingredients and use over salads, including fruit salad.

Rich English Dressing (adrenal, muscular, thyroid)

2 yolks of organic eggs
½ cup lemon juice
1 can thick unsweetened milk
¼ cup organic butter
1 teaspoon mustard
1 teaspoon sea salt or Herbamere

Melt butter and set aside. Add egg yolks to a bowl and add milk, stirring constantly. Add lemon juice, mustard, and salt (or Herbamere), then melted butter. Set aside to allow to stiffen; place in a covered jar and refrigerate. Use with any vegetable or meat dish.

Parsley Butter (adrenal, thyroid, muscular)

3 oz. organic butter
1 T. chopped fresh parsley
juice ½ lemon
sea salt to taste

Soften butter and on a plate with a wooden spoon stir in gradually all remaining ingredients. Serve over grilled steaks, liver, kidneys, and fish or atop a baked potato.

Make-Your-Own Salted Almonds (all types, especially adrenal)

½ pound good quality organic almonds

fine sea salt

1 T. organic butter or 2 T. extra virgin olive oil (or for a real treat 2 or 3
   T. Poppy Seed Oil)

Place almonds in a bowl. Cover with boiling water. Let stand for 5 to
6 minutes. Throw into cold water, then immediately remove skin with
fingers. To skin simply take almond between the right thumb and the
first finger, and rub off the skin. Dry with a towel. Put the butter or oil
in a flat baking tin and the prepared nuts, and put them in a medium
oven, stirring every 8 minutes, until they are nicely browned and have
absorbed most of the fat. When ready, move with a spoon to a dish
lined with brown paper or brown paper towels. Sprinkle heavily with
salt and a dash of paprika and/or curry powder. Shake off any loose
salt, and turn on to another piece of brown paper to dry. Store, until
cold, in an airtight glass jar. Serve in a fine crystal or clear glass
compote or nice stem glass.

Avocado Cream Dressing (thyroid, pituitary)

1 cup avocado pulp

large pinch sea salt

2 T. Wild Oregano Honey or Thistle Honey

1 cup organic heavy cream

teaspoon Raw Wild Blackberry Extract (optional)

Rub avocado through sieve or fruit press. Add salt, blackberry extract,
and honey; mix thoroughly. Whip cream and fold in avocado pulp. Serve
over any salad, especially fruit salad.

Drinks and Smoothies

Certain nutrients in high concentrations can greatly aid adrenal types. Because of their high rate of metabolism they require great quantities of nutrients. They can achieve this through the fruit-based smoothies and juices. However, there is a caveat: they must avoid excessive intake of fruit and particularly excessive quantities of highly sweet juice, such as commercial apple, pear, grape, and orange juice and particularly excessive amounts of vegetable juices. When drinking vegetable juices, they must always be salted. This includes carrot juice.

Simple Lemon-Lime Juice with Raw Honey (thyroid, adrenal, muscular)

2 organic lemons, juiced, seeds removed
2 organic limes, juiced, seeds removed
2 T. Wild Oregano Honey (or Canadian Wild Flower Honey)

Mix all ingredients and drink for morning cleansing. Or, chill and serve with meals.

Pomegranate Sour 'Lemonade' (all types)

2 quarts pure water
dozen ice cubes
7 T. Sour Mediterranean Pomegranate Extract
juice of 2 lemons (optional)

Mix and serve immediately or chill and serve later. If desired, serve with fresh mint leaves. Or, add fresh mint leaves and let chill to give added flavor and then serve. May also substitute sparkling mineral water.

Carob and Yogurt Cream Shake (adrenal, muscular, pituitary)

2 T. Wild Carob Concentrate (Car-o-Power)
1 or more cups full-fat organic yogurt
handful pine nuts or blanched almonds
cold water and/or ice

In a blender blend all ingredients, adding water/ice to desired thickness.
Ideal for children.

Maca Root Adrenal Coffee (adrenal, thyroid)

1 level T. MacaPunch Xpresso
2 T. heavy cream
2 or 3 cups pure water

Heat water to a boil and add MacaPunch and heavy cream. Drink as a
calming and nourishing beverage. Note: the maca is grainy and so it
won't completely dissolve. Alternatively, put all ingredients in a blender
and whip for a few moments and then serve.

Carob Milk (adrenal, muscular)

4 T. Car-o-Power
quart whole organic milk
handful pine nuts or blanched almonds (optional)
1 T. Organic Rice Bran (optional)

In a blender blend until fully blended. For energy, drink immediately.

Clean-You-Out Wild Berry Smoothie (all types)

cup wild berries, your choice
cup or more full-fat organic yogurt

2 T. Liquid Wild Berry Extract (Raw 8 Berry Extract; dried berry
   extracts are too weak)

few pine nuts or blanched almonds

2 T. Wild Oregano Honey or Mediterranean Wild Flower Honey optional
   but very cleansing)

ice or water to desired thickness

In a blender mix to desired thickness. Makes an ideal breakfast. For
people with constipation add a tablespoon Wild Carob Concentrate. The
latter is a gentle stool softener.

Berried Almond Milk Smoothie (mainly pituitary but also adrenal)

1 or 2 cups almond milk

1 tablespoon raw wild oregano honey

2 tablespoons organic rice bran

1 organic or free-range egg yolk

blueberries or papaya (for color and taste)

teaspoon Wild Raw Blackberry Extract or Wild Raw Huckleberry Extract

cold water (as needed)

In a blender blend until smooth, adding fruit and water to desired
thickness. Drink as a full breakfast, supper, or lunch. The eggs provide
zinc, direly needed by the thyroid gland, as well as the muscular system,
while the rice bran provides thiamine and niacin, which are required for
hormone production. The milk and/or almond milk provides calcium,
magnesium, and riboflavin.

Mostly Adrenal Smoothie (adrenal and muscular)

contents of three capsules royal jelly (undiluted, triple-X)

3 T. Rice Polish/Bran/Crushed Flax Combination

1 cup or more whole organic milk

1 cup combination of strawberries and/or blueberries

1 to 2 organic or farm raised egg yolk, raw (mix in a drop of oil of wild oregano to kill any bacteria)

2 T. Wild Oregano Honey

In a blender blend until smooth, adding water to desired thickness. Drink as an addition to breakfast or as a complete meal.

Proper Adrenal Carrot Juice (adrenal and muscular)

1 quart organic carrot juice

1/3 teaspoon sea salt

2 T. organic heavy cream

1 T. Organic Rice Bran

ice

In a blender blend until frothy.

Super-Thyroid Smoothie (thyroid and possibly adrenal)

handful pine nuts

1 pint or more whole organic milk

large handful organic strawberries or blueberries

3 T. Organic Rice Bran or mixture of Rice Bran, Rice Polish, Ground Flax, and Red Sour Grape

Blend all ingredients until smooth. Add water to desired thickness, if necessary. Add a few ice cubes for a chilled taste.

Pituitary-Power Smoothie (pituitary)

handful pine nuts or blanched almonds

1 pint rice or almond milk

3 T. Purely Natural B Complex powder

large handful organic blueberries

1 T. Wild Oregano Honey

1-2 T. Organically grown Hand-Picked Sacha Inchi or Raw Multi-Seed
Oil

Blend all ingredients until smooth, adding water or ice, if desired.

Muscle-Freak Smoothie (muscular, adrenal)

handful blanched almonds

1 pint whole organic milk

2 T. Multi-Seed Oil or Remote-Source Poppy Seed Oil (the latter is rich
in pre-hormones)

2 teaspoons Red Sour Grape Powder

yolk of one organic egg (optional; add a drop or two of oil of wild
oregano to the yolk and mix)

3 T. Organic Rice Bran or mixture of Rice Bran, Rice Polish, Ground
Flax, and Red Sour Grape

ice or water, as needed

Blend all ingredients until smooth, adding water or ice to desired thickness.

Tropical Rice Bran Smoothie (pituitary)

1 avocado, peeled and seeded

1 mango, seeded

3 heaping T. Organic Rice Bran or Rice Bran, torula yeast, and royal jelly
(Purely Natural B Complex powder)

raw honey as needed (optional)

handful pine nuts or blanched almonds (makes it creamier)

ice and water as needed

In a blender or VitaMix process to desired thickness. Freeze as an ice cream. Have solely as a nutritious breakfast.

Tropical Rice Bran Smoothie with Full Fat Yogurt (all types)

1 cup or more full fat organic yogurt

1 mango, seeded

3 heaping T. Organic Rice Bran or preferably a Rice Bran/Polish/Crushed Flax Mix

1 teaspoon Red Sour Grape Powder (chromium-rich)

handful pine nuts or blanched almonds (makes it creamier, optional)

ice and water as needed

In a blender blend to desired thickness. Freeze as an ice cream. Have solely as a nutritious breakfast.

Special High-Powered Citrus Juice (mainly adrenal but also muscular)

This juice is ideal for adrenal types, because of the great need for vitamin C, required for adrenal steroid synthesis. This should be consumed regularly to ensure ideal vitamin C intake.

2 organic oranges, cut in halves

1 organic grapefruit, halved

1 organic lemon, halved

Remove seeds as much as possible and juice. Drink immediately. Optional: add honey and freeze as a special treat. Note: when juicing, try to grind out as much of the inner white pulp as possible, as this pulp is high in bioflavonoids. The latter help in the regeneration of connective tissue, skin, and blood vessels.

Mixed Berries in Whole Fat Milk (mainly adrenal but also pituitary, if using blueberries)

Whole fat milk (ideally, raw unpasteurized and unhomogenized)
Mixture of organic berries, ideally blueberries and strawberries)

Add berries to a bowl and pour half or more cup of milk. Enjoy as a snack or dessert.

Note: for pituitary types make a nut milk from pine nuts and blanched almonds; pour over the berries and enjoy.

'Cocoa'-Like Almond Shake (adrenal, muscular, pituitary)

3 T. Wild Carob Concentrate (Car-o-Power)
1 cup blanched almonds
3 T. pine nuts
1 or 2 T. Rice Polish, Rice Bran, Crushed Flax, and Red Sour Grape
Mix ice and water to desired thickness

Blend well, and serve chilled.

Natural Blueberry Milk Shake (adrenal and pituitary)

handful organic blueberries
whole organic milk
combination Rice Polish, Rice Bran, Crushed Flax
a few blanched almonds and/or pine nuts

Blend all ingredients to desired thickness and content.

Endocrine note: Rice bran/polish provides a dense supply of B vitamins, which the hormone glands need for synthesis. Pituitary and adrenal function are greatly improved through natural B vitamins. The fat in the milk aids the absorption of the berry flavonoids. These berry flavonoids have hormone-like actions.

Special Fruit Juice (all types)

Note: this is an ideal juice for people with thyroid conditions. It is relatively low in sugar, so it is also good for the adrenal types. Blueberries are helpful for pituitary types. Papayas are ideal for muscular types. So, this is universal juice. In general, vegetable juices contain goitrogens, which stall thyroid function. Thus, this juice emphasizes fruit. To spice it up a bit of unbleached sea salt is added, a source of iodine.

$\frac{1}{2}$ to 1 cup blueberries, washed (or use frozen organic variety; let thaw)
$\frac{1}{2}$ papaya, seeded and peeled
2 kiwi fruit
2 teaspoons Wild Raw Huckleberry Extract (limited supply, rare)
sea salt

Juice; add sea salt to taste and drink immediately.

Salty Vegetable Juice (thyroid)

Certain vegetables are relatively low in goitrogens. This juice emphasizes those vegetables. Crude sea salt is added both for taste as well as a source of iodine. For added power Special High Quality Ground Kelp (GreenBay Naturally Wild) may be added. Kelp and seasalt neutralize any goitrogenic effects.

4 fresh organic tomatoes, quartered
2 small zucchini (a natural source of salt)
celery (a natural source of salt)
ground kelp or other dried seaweed (or three capsules of a crude kelp
    complex of northern Pacific and northern Atlantic source)

Juice; then, add sea salt and kelp (or capsules). Let sit for several hours while refrigerated and then drink.

Desserts

There is no need for a large number of desserts. The meals are satisfying on their own. In fact, the smoothies act as desserts. Regardless, here are a few examples for healthy eating:

Berries and Caroby Cream (all types)

1 cup organic blueberries
1 cup organic strawberries, sliced
1/3 cup organic raspberries
pint organic cream
2 T. Wild Carob Concentrate (Car-o-Power)

Whip cream and Carob Molasses; chill. Mix berries and cover with cream; serve cold.

Healthy Marzipan (adrenal, muscular)

1/2 pound ground almonds
1/2 pound unprocessed honey
a few Brazil nuts
1 or 2 organic eggs
2 teaspoons Mediterranean Grape Concentrate (Grape-o-Power)

With a rolling pin grind almonds and Brazil nuts. In a bowl add nuts and honey. Make a hollow in the center with the back of a wooden spoon; drop in eggs and grape concentrate. Mix to a stiff paste and serve.

Berries in Milk with Organic Rice Bran (all types)

Rice bran is rich in the B vitamins needed for processing sugars. It is also rich in chromium, also needed for the metabolism of sugar, including fruit sugar.

organic milk (or rice milk)
1 cup organic blueberries or blackberries
1 cup organic strawberries, sliced
a few raspberries (optional)
1 or 2 T. Organic Rice Bran
2 T. Wild Unprocessed Raw Honey (ideally, Wild Oregano Honey)

Add berries to bowl; drizzle with honey and add rice bran. Pour in milk or eat with rice milk.

Peach and Nectarine Delight (adrenal, muscular)

4 organic peaches
4 organic nectarines
2 T. Mediterranean grape concentrate (Grape-o-Power)
3 T. organic heavy cream
T. Organic Rice Bran or Combination Rice Bran, Rice Polish, and
    Crushed Flax (optional)

Wash peaches and nectarines. Cut into slices. Arrange on plate; drizzle with grape concentrate and heavy cream; also top with rice bran or Nutri-Sense (Note: do not use commercial grape concentrate, as it is too refined and unhealthy; use only the true Mediterranean type).

Orange-Walnut Fruit Salad (pituitary, thyroid)

3 oranges, peeled, sectioned, and chopped
1 grapefruit, peeled, seeded, sectioned, and chopped
a bit of lime juice
2 tangerines, peeled, sectioned
handful or two of walnuts

Mix all ingredients in a bowl and toss. Serve chilled.

Endocrine note: walnuts are rich in omega-3 fatty acids, desperately needed by the pituitary as well as the thyroid gland. To make this an ideal adrenal or muscular recipe simply pour over whole organic milk or cream.

Ideal Snacks

The following is a list of snacks that are ideal between meals. Also, they make perfect travel snacks to prevent disrupting any metabolic gains, that is by succumbing to temptation and eating processed foods. These snacks are listed by body type.

Ideal snacks for pituitary types: Dark Austrian Pumpkin Seeds, Sprouted Organic Pumpkin seeds, Sprouted Organic Sunflower Seeds, Dry Roasted Sprouted Salted Almonds, Artichokes in Extra Virgin Olive Oil, Cherry Tomatoes in Extra Virgin Olive Oil, Natural Basil Pesto Sauce (without cheese), dried fish, sardines, dried blueberries (or fresh), dried strawberries, filberts, pecans, walnuts, pine nuts, Wild remote-source Sockeye Salmon (canned or vacuum-packed), wild or remote-source Dried Saskatoon Berries.

Ideal snacks for adrenal types: Sliced salted roast beef or turkey, chicken wings or drumsticks (salted), Sprouted Nuts of all types, especially Almonds and Sunflower Seeds as well as Pistachios. Natural Olive Paste, Natural Sun-dried Tomato Paste, Natural Sun-dried Tomatoes, Pesto Sauce with Cheese, Sugar-Free Turkey or Beef Jerky, (raw honey is OK), dried blueberries, dried strawberries, dry roasted salted organic peanuts, salted almonds, salted filberts, salted pistachios, pine nuts, Natural Olive Paste, natural grass-fed Bison jerky (no sugar added; nitrate-free), Wild Remote-Source Sockeye Salmon (canned or vacuum-packed).

-

Ideal snacks for thyroid types: Sliced roast turkey or beef, chicken wings or drumsticks, whole fat yogurt, Sprouted Pistachios, Sprouted Sunflower Seeds, Sprouted Almonds, Olives, Artichokes in Extra Virgin Olive Oil, Sugar-Free Turkey or Beef Jerky, Bison Jerky, dried strawberries (or fresh), dried blueberries (or fresh), walnuts, filberts, pine nuts, Brazil nuts, Natural Basil Pesto (with or without cheese), Natural Sun-dried Tomato Paste, Natural Sun-dried Tomatoes, Natural Olive Paste, Natural Grass-Fed Bison Jerky (no sugar added; nitrate-free), Wild Remote-Source Sockeye Salmon (canned or vacuum-packed).

Ideal snacks for muscular types: sprouted nuts of all types, remote-source raisins (such as Monuka raisins) for energy, dried mulberries, flax bread, dates (small quantities), sugar-free Turkey or Beef Jerky, Bison Jerky, pickled eggs, gently smoked fish, Wild Remote-Source Sockeye Salmon (canned or vacuum-packed).

Note: many of these foods are available at Americanwildfoods.com. Shop at this site for better health. Here, the food is superior and more unique than what is found anywhere in the world. Remember, all items capitalized are specialty items available on this site.

Chapter Twelve
Conclusion

The human body reveals its own patterns. The shape gives the ultimate clue. Obviously, the body is controlled by higher forces. Perhaps humans don't always understand these forces. Before the publication of this book no one knew that the body attempted to give signals of its true nature. It does so, even by its bone structure and shape, even by the length of the fingers. This is what the endocrine system reveals. Let people heed it. As a result, spectacular health can be achieved. Let them give it credence to avoid catastrophes—the catastrophes of preventable illness and premature death.

Now, it is time to be grateful to the high creator. He has created a system, which is obvious. It is written on a person's face, in their skeleton and musculature, in their hands, and even in their abdomens. It is all available for humans to use, if they will just take advantage of it. In a mere minute or less a person can determine his/her type. This is a blessing.

It is incredible, but every person is different. The nature of a person's physiology is revealed through external features. The system is easy to understand and easy to apply. Once this code is revealed, then, the exact treatment can be dispensed. This will free humans of the burden of illness. The endocrine glands are the main source of this uniqueness. These glands control metabolism. The metabolism controls all functions. These functions include circulation, digestion, muscular activity, the strengthening of the bones, elimination, lymph flow, and energy. Thus, the monumental nature of the metabolic type is obvious.

Most people are in poor health. Or, they lack vitality. Discovering the endocrine type is the key link to regenerating this. This is the person's opportunity to easily improve health. In fact, improvement literally occurs overnight. It is even essential to longevity. Again, if the metabolism is dysfunctional, all body systems are faulty. When the endocrine system is disturbed, none of the organs can function adequately. Thus, the importance of determining the endocrine type and taking the appropriate treatment is made clear.

This must also be the focus of those with chronic illnesses. These are the people who suffer endlessly from health conditions, with no answers. They are the individuals who may well have lost hope, since no one was able to determine the underlying factors and therefore reverse the condition. Thus, they must take the metabolic type challenge and follow the advise. This is because it is the endocrine status which determines the inner workings of the body, including the metabolism. What's more, the metabolism determines the key issue: how a person's cells and organs function as well as thrive on a daily basis. The metabolic type also determines diet and nutritional needs. It also reveals the exact course of treatment for reversing the condition and also preventing further disease.

Now, the needs of the body can be accurately addressed. This is based upon an inherent type, which is built within the individual. The type fits into the pattern that acts as a guide. These are mainly the thyroid, adrenal, pituitary, thyroid-adrenal, and adrenal-thyroid types. There are also the two subtypes, the thyroid-muscular and the adrenal-pituitary. Now, the proper therapy can be prescribed. The healing process can also be efficiently stimulated. The entire symphony of the body can be put into balance. As a result, the body can be kept in the most ideal health possible.

The pattern is definite. There are the thyroid types, who are often rectangular- or square-shaped and who often have square-shaped heads. They have the fat—if they are overweight—on the front of the body, from the chest down but mainly in the front of the abdomen and the front of the thighs. The buttocks are usually flattened, although in some instances there may be fat deposition in the form of cellulite. There may also be cellulite along the outside of the thighs. The ankles are often swollen, as are the hands. With a pure thyroid type there is not much curvature to the hips; most of any excess weight is centered in the front of the abdomen and thighs. If there is curvature along the hips, it means there is a pituitary component. The so-called love handles, those creases of sagging tissue along the mid- to low-back are typical. Also, in this type the tissues may be swollen. They are often puffy all over, and there is often swelling under and over the eyes. The eyelids may also be swollen. Usually, the fingers are also puffy. In extreme cases the skin of the face is thickened. The hair is also usually coarse or thick. Also, a droopy-appearing face is typical of this type. In particular, the corners of the eyes and mouth droop downward.

The hands in the thyroid type are characteristic. Very long fingers and palms are rare. Often, the hands are stubby or medium in length. Occasionally, the fingers are medium- to long. However, most characteristic is a short (normal) first finger compared to the fourth finger, that is the index finger is shorter than the ring. Usually, there is much ridging on the nails, especially in extreme cases. The hair on the head is often thick, although in extreme cases there is major hair loss from the scalp, especially in women. There may also be hair loss along the outer third of the eyebrows. Other characteristics and symptoms are mentioned throughout this book.

The adrenal type is usually thin. Even so, with this type moderate obesity can occur. The bone structure is often fine but not always. Yet, they still usually have delicate features, at least more delicate than the thyroid type. More importantly, the facial bones are thin. The person with the typical receding chin or a person with thin jaw bones is the adrenal type. Usually, the face is more angular and less square than the thyroid type. The skin on the face is also more thin than is skin in thyroid types. The hair is thin to medium.

In adrenal types since the bones of the face are abnormally small there are major dental problems. Often, with this type there is crowding of the lower incisors. There may also be impaction of the wisdom teeth. Crowding of both the upper and lower incisors is a sign of extreme adrenal exhaustion. This may also be seen combination types.

Weight is often held in the buttocks but not grossly so. In women adrenal types simply have better curvature here than the thyroid type. There may be a pouch of weight or fluid located just below the umbilicus, known medically as visceroptosis. The latter means drooping of the viscera or internal organs. Also, adrenal types often have thin hair on their arms and legs. The typically flat-chested female is an adrenal type.

The hands, particularly the fingers, are characteristic. Usually, the first finger is longer or as long as the ring finger. A long index finger is relatively rare, discovered in no more than one of ten people. For further information check the diagrams of this book. Like the thyroid type there are typical hair distribution patterns. Again, the hair on the scalp is usually exceptionally fine, although in the thyroid-adrenal type it may be medium-fine. It is rarely coarse. There is typically sparse hair on the rest of the body, especially the thighs and legs. There is also often hair loss on the lower third of the outer leg (below the knees). The blond and blue-eyed person with fine hair is the classic example of the adrenal type. Even so, the important point is that adrenal types are those who have a propensity for weak adrenal function.

Obviously, thyroid-adrenal types are a combination of these patterns. One characteristic feature is the fact that these types usually have a combination of the hand-finger signs. In other words, one hand has a long or equal index finger compared to the ring, while the other is the opposite. The way to determine this (in a person whose fingernails are short) is to place the hands in a relaxed way palm down with the fingers together on a piece of paper. Then, draw the outline with a pencil. Using a ruler draw a straight line between the top of the outline of the fingers by placing the edge of the ruler on the shortest finger (that is which ever is shortest, the ring or the index).

360 The Body Shape Diet

The pituitary type is more rare. Yet, there are pituitary components within many of the other types. With the pituitary type there are two variations. The most common is the anterior pituitary type, corresponding to the anterior pituitary gland. This one predominates. Here, the face or rather head is small compared to the body size. So are the hands and feet. The body is pear shaped, with the excess weight being held in the hips, buttocks, and lateral thighs. The shoulders may be tiny. If there is a thyroid component, the buttocks may be flattened but otherwise they are plump.

The hands are often puffy. There is often a combination of finger signs as mentioned previously, with one index finger being longer than the ring and on the other side the opposite.

The head/face may also be characteristic. Often, it is circular or even moon-shaped. In fact, in such people the entire body can be rotund. The center of the abdomen may also have a rounded appearance. Here, too, for the size of the body the head may appear small. There may also be sagging of the back of the arms and, too, the ankles may be large. In addition, the entire body may appear swollen, with the swelling existing in the face, neck, middle abdomen, and outer thighs. Such people have extreme difficulty losing weight, yet they do so readily on this endocrine plan. Often, in these types, like the thyroid-adrenal, one hand will exhibit a long index finger compared to the ring and the other will be opposite. Or, the fingers may be a bit stubby and both fingers are about the same length on both hands. The hands and feet are tiny compared to the rest of the body. This is a key sign of this type. Yet, there are variations. Even so, it is the pattern which is critical.

In the more rare variation, which is the posterior pituitary type, the hands are long, as are the fingers. The head is large, as are the feet.

Those with the muscular component have the appearance of a coach, weight lifter, or, perhaps, marathon runner. They are sturdy and strong. The are well muscled, even if they don't exercise. One characteristic component is large calves and well muscled thighs. If they do carry weight, it is in the front of the abdomen. Often, they have a short chest cage and large lungs. This may explain why they can maintain such powerful muscles. An interesting note is that these persons often crave alcohol and may be heavy drinkers. A short-to-medium boxy body shape is typical of this type. A variant is a long rectangular chest cage, again with hefty lungs.

It is the endocrine glands which create these differences. The cells are mere end organs. Large organs, like the liver, spleen, intestines, and brain, are also end organs. In other words, they are unable to determine their own fate. It is the hormone system which controls these. Cells are merely mechanical adjuncts, mere end organs operating to serve the higher element. The true control arises in the nervous system, that is the brain and spinal cord. In turn, the hormones directly influence the function capacity of the brain and nerves. The nervous system delivers messages to the endocrine glands, which produce the secretions necessary to maintain life. So, in fact, all control ultimately arises through these glands. These glands are influenced by thoughts. Positive thoughts positively influence them. In contrast, negative thoughts disrupt them. Furthermore, prayer to the almighty creator is a powerful therapy, since it helps calm the glands. The human being finds great peace in prayer. This, then, positively influences glandular function. In contrast, despair and anger inflame the glandular system.

The importance of such glands over all other organs is readily demonstrated. For instance, consider other crucial organs which do not secrete endocrine substances: the spleen, appendix, colon, stomach, thymus, and lymph nodes. All can be removed, and life will continue. Not so with the key endocrine glands. Remove any, and life will either cease or existence will be reduced to mere despair. For instance, if all parathyroid glands are removed, rapidly, death ensues. The same is true of the adrenals and to a degree thyroid. If the pituitary is removed, the patient may survive but only poorly. If the ovaries or testes are removed, there will be survival, but overall health will greatly decline.

So, obviously, human life is dependent upon the glands. Thus, for improvement to rapidly occur—for the healthy to be revitalized—the endocrine system must be strengthened and balanced. Consider heart disease. Here, the emphasis of the medical profession has always been on the heart muscle itself. This is erroneous. Instead, the thyroid, and adrenals, as well as the liver, and sex glands should be the focus. If this was the case, if these glands were systematically strengthened, virtually all heart disease could be cured, that is without doing anything specific for the heart. No angiograms, angioplasty, cardiograms, stress test, cardiac drugs, or by-pass surgery: merely by correcting the metabolic defect, the problem is solved.

Imagine the value of such a system. Millions of lives would be saved, and untold pain and agony avoided. Imagine the financial savings. It would be untold billions of dollars yearly. For liver disease the emphasis has always been on this organ. True, there are other key issues. For instance, the various functions of digestion and elimination are crucial as is the health of the great organ of detoxification, the liver. Yet, merely focusing on the liver, colon, and kidneys is insufficient. Actually, the functions of these organs is largely controlled by the hormone system. So, it is paramount for cleaning and healing the body to support the function of the glands.

For cancer the immune system is managed by the adrenal glands, thymus, and thyroid gland. So, in the treatment of this disease to focus only on the immune cells would be a mistake. For high blood pressure the adrenal glands, as well as the thyroid, play a major role. With diabetes the emphasis has been on the pancreas, when the greater role is played by all the other hormonal organs, that is the organs of metabolism such as the liver, adrenal glands, pituitary, and thyroid. In arthritis the adrenal glands play a predominant role, since they control the process of inflammation. Yet, the thyroid also plays a role, since it masters the balance of proper circulation to the muscles and joints.

Regarding mental diseases the emphasis has been exclusively upon the brain. Yet, this organ is of minor importance, that is compared to the benefit of supporting the pituitary, thyroid, and adrenals. In digestive disorders, for instance, hiatus hernia, ulcers, and gastric reflux, the emphasis has been on the stomach and intestines directly, when it is the adrenal glands and thyroid gland which balance the digestive process. It is these organs which must be treated first before any treatment of the gut is considered. With thyroid disorders the stress has always been on this organ alone. Yet, there should also be emphasis upon the pituitary and in many instances ovaries and adrenal glands.

It becomes obvious that regarding the endocrine system medicine has failed. What's more, regarding the treatment of actual diseases—heart disease, cancer, autoimmune disorders, hepatitis, lung disease, kidney disease, hypo- or hyperthyroidism, adrenal disorders, diabetes, mental diseases, and arthritis—there is no success. This failure is due to a simple fact, which is the neglect to treat the cause.

The endocrine type is the same as the metabolic type. The metabolism is under hormonal control. Hormones, the secretions of the glands, drive the metabolism. Call it the endocrine type, hormone type, body type, body shape type—whatever it is called it all means the same, which is that it is that system which controls how a person feels, metabolizes, digests, and survives. It is that system which manifests a person's strengths and accounts for any weaknesses.

The metabolic type is a reliable solution for health improvement. Through this system a person's health can be revitalized virtually immediately. The purpose is to find the cause of all illness, and prescribe the correct treatment. With this system the treatment is based upon the exact cause, as determined by the metabolic type. All people have a type. For each person the secret is to discover the exact type so overall health can be improved. It is also so that disease can be aggressively reversed. This is the metabolic promise, which is that the individual can get well through a systematic approach that is individualized and accurate.

Based on the shape of the body the metabolic type is the key to perfect health. This shows the way to the real nature of a person's body. Now, superb health is easy to achieve. There is nothing in medicine so fascinating or so reliable as this type. It is the true window into the function of the body for every person. So, now a person's health can be dramatically improved. This is also the tool to *keep* the body healthy. Too, it is the means to gain as much power and stamina as possible. A person will feel more internally vibrant on this plan. As well, it is that key element for perhaps lengthening life span. That is the body shape type guarantee.

Appendix A

The following is a summary of the various food supplements recommended for each type. It represents a general or basic protocol for rebuilding and strengthening the endocrine system. Other recommendations are found throughout this book.

This describes high-quality brands, which exist in superior health food stores. These brands are also available for purchase on the internet. There are also internet sources in England and the Netherlands, which service Europe and Asia (see oliveleaf.co.uk and vivanatura.nl). Quality health food stores in the United States either stock these items or may order them. In Ireland health food stores are well stocked with these supplements. In England NutriCentre is another source. Supplements are listed in order of priority. Some people may choose to start with those listed as first priority, adding others later.

Food supplements for the thyroid type

1st Priority

- Crude rice bran/polish powder with crushed sprouted flax-seed and red sour grape (the latter being a high chromium source); Also, natural source whole food B complex supplement made from torula yeast, rice bran, and royal jelly

- Wild kelp-based supplement with crude wild oregano and tyrosine, the kelp being derived from northern Pacific and northern Atlantic sources

- Natural-source vitamin C, as a combination of camu camu, acerola, and rose hips

- Natural-source riboflavin (from wild raw greens drops and drinks)

- Mediterranean-source oil of wild oregano from hand-picked wild spice (for purging fungi and viruses)

- Wild oregano crude herb (as capsules with *Rhus coriaria*)

2nd priority

- Natural-source zinc (from pumpkinseeds, meat, and fish—there is no natural-source zinc pill, although wild oregano capsules contain homeopathic-like doses)

- Special purging agent with wild raw greens, raw apple cider vinegar, raw black seed oil, spice oils, and extra virgin olive oil

- Natural-source chromium (from red sour grape)

- Wild raw 8 berries complex (northern Canada source)

- Special digestive enzyme complex with non-GM enzymes plus papain and bromelain, along with potent spice extracts, including fenugreek and cardamom

- Fatty wild sockeye salmon oil, polar source, with rich amounts of vitamins A and D

3rd priority

- Natural organically grown Peruvian inca nut (sacha inchi) oil

- Multiple spice extract (for syndrome X; this complex eliminates insulin resistance)

- Wild chaga mushroom extract (as emulsified drops under the tongue with wild oregano or expresso with wild birch bark)

- High-grade Mediterranean sour pomegranate concentrate

Note: an all-in-one thyroid support supplement is now available (Body Shape Plan; thyroid support). This supplement contains many of the key substances needed by the thyroid type, all in one bottle.

Food supplements for the adrenal type

1st priority

- Undiluted 3x royal jelly fortified with adrenal-strengthening herbs (rosemary and sage)

- Raw royal jelly paste, ideally emulsified in essential oils and crude, cold-pressed, dark green pumpkinseed oil

- Natural-source vitamin C, as a combination of camu camu, acerola, and rose hips

- Wild triple salt capsules with wild rosemary and oregano

- Crude, unprocessed maca powder and/or original maca raw beverage (undiluted) and maca coffee (to strengthen the adrenal glands—contain adrenal-like hormones); this is remote Andean source, available at Americanwildfoods.com

- Mediterranean-source oil of wild oregano from the hand-picked wild spice (for purging fungi)

- Wild chaga mushroom extract (as emulsified drops under the tongue with wild oregano or expresso with wild birch bark)

2nd priority

- Crude, organic rice bran or rice bran/polish powder with crushed flax and red sour grape (the latter a high-chromium source)

- Raw crude Austrian-source pumpkinseed oil (as a source of hormones and pre-hormones)

- Spice combination for healthy female hormone function (for women with correspondingly weak ovaries)—fennel, fenugreek, sage, and royal jelly

- Multiple spice complex extract (for regulating blood sugar and eliminating sugar cravings; eliminates insulin resistance)

- Oil of wild rosemary (and its water essence or juice)

- Salt grass

Note: an all-in-one adrenal support supplement is now available (Body Shape Plan; adrenal support). This supplement contains many of the key substances needed by the adrenal type, all in one bottle.

Food supplements for the thyroid-adrenal type (also use this protocol for adrenal-thyroid)

1st Priority

- Crude rice bran/polish powder with crushed sprouted flaxseed and red sour grape (the latter being a high chromium source), or natural source whole food B complex supplement made from torula yeast, rice bran, and royal jelly

- Wild kelp-based supplement with crude wild oregano and

tyrosine, the kelp being derived from northern Pacific and northern Atlantic sources

- Natural-source vitamin C, as a combination of camu camu, acerola, and rose hips

- Natural-source riboflavin (from wild greens drops and drinks)

- Mediterranean-source oil of wild oregano from hand-picked wild spice (for purging fungi and viruses)

- Wild oregano crude herb (as capsules with *Rhus coriaria*)

- Undiluted 3x royal jelly fortified with adrenal strengthening herbs (rosemary and sage)

- Raw royal jelly paste, ideally emulsified in essential oils and crude, cold-pressed, dark green pumpkinseed oil

2nd priority

- Special purging agent with wild raw greens, raw apple cider vinegar, raw black seed oil, spice oils, and extra virgin olive oil

- Spice combination for healthy female hormone function (for women with correspondingly weak ovaries)—fennel, fenugreek, sage, and royal jelly

- Wild, raw 8-berries complex

- Special digestive enzyme complex with non-GM enzymes plus papain and bromelain, along with potent spice extracts, including fenugreek and cardamom

- Fatty wild sockeye salmon oil, polar source, with rich amounts of vitamins A and D

- Salt grass

3rd priority

- Natural organically grown Peruvian inca nut (sacha inchi) oil

- Multiple spice extract (for syndrome X; this complex eliminates insulin resistance)

- Wild chaga mushroom extract (as emulsified drops under the tongue with wild oregano or expresso with wild birch bark)

- Wild triple salt capsules with wild rosemary and oregano

- Crude, unprocessed maca powder and/or original maca raw beverage (undiluted) and maca coffee (to strengthen the adrenal glands—contain adrenal-like hormones); this is remote Andean source, available at Americanwildfoods.com

- Mediterranean-source oil of wild oregano

Food supplements for the pituitary type

1st priority

- Crude rice bran/polish powder with crushed sprouted flaxseed and red sour grape (the latter being a high chromium source) or natural source whole food B complex supplement made from torula yeast, rice bran, and royal jelly

- Natural wild plant-source omega-3s, as organically-grown sacha inchi oil

- Fatty wild sockeye salmon oil, polar source, with rich amounts of vitamins A and D

- Wild greens drops and/or wild nettle juice

- natural-source vitamin C, as a combination of camu camu, acerola, and rose hips

- Raw royal jelly paste, ideally emulsified in essential oils and crude cold-pressed dark green pumpkinseed oil

- Crude unprocessed maca root powder or preferably liquid extract and/or maca coffee (as ground roasted maca root)

- Wild, raw berries complex (8 wild berry mix)

- Spice combination for healthy female hormone function (for women with correspondingly weak ovaries)—fennel, fenugreek, Sage, and Royal Jelly

- Mediterranean-source oil of wild oregano from hand-picked wild spice (for purging fungi)

2nd priority

- Wild huckleberry and/or blueberry extract

- Multiple spice extract, especially for those with heavy hips (for regulating blood sugar and eliminating sugar cravings; also, this complex eliminates insulin resistance)

- Red sour grape (as a source of blood sugar-regulating chromium)

- Oil of wild rosemary (and its water-essence or juice)

- Natural purging agent (wild greens, plus spice oils) for heavy metal overload.

- Special digestive enzyme complex with non-GM enzymes plus papain and bromelain, along with potent spice extracts

Note: an all-in-one pituitary support supplement is now available (Body Shape Plan; pituitary support). This supplement contains many of the key substances needed by the pituitary type, all in one bottle.　　　　ₗ'I

Food supplements for thyroid-muscular (muscular-pancreatic) type

1st priority

• Natural-source whole food B complex supplement made from torula yeast, rice bran, and royal jelly

• Special digestive enzyme complex with non-GM enzymes plus papain and bromelain, along with potent spice extracts

• Red sour grape (as a source of muscle-building chromium and sour flavonoids)

• taurine (as amino acid chelate)

• magnesium (as amino acid chelate)

• Crude wild oregano herb (as capsules with *Rhus coriaria*)

• Wild greens drops containing wild dandelion, burdock, and nettles and/or wild super-5 greens juice

2nd priority

• Special liver-cleansing capsules with wild raw dandelion leaf, cumin, and turmeric

• Special purging agent with wild raw greens, raw apple cider vinegar, raw black seed oil, spice oils, and extra virgin olive oil

- Wild chaga mushroom extract (as emulsified drops under the tongue with wild oregano or expresso with wild birch bark)

Food supplements for the pituitary-thyroid-adrenal type

1st priority

- Natural-source vitamin C, as a combination of camu camu, acerola, and rose hips

- Special purging agent with wild raw greens, raw apple cider vinegar, raw black seed oil, spice oils, and extra virgin olive oil

- Crude organic rice bran/polish powder with crushed flax and red sour grape (the latter a high chromium source)

- Undiluted 3x royal jelly fortified with adrenal strengthening herbs (rosemary and sage)

- Wild raw berries complex (8 wild berry mix)

2nd priority

- Spice combination for healthy female hormone function (for women with correspondingly weak ovaries)—fennel, fenugreek, sage, and royal jelly

- Unprocessed yacon syrup (remote Andean source) for balancing blood sugar

- Raw royal jelly paste, ideally emulsified in essential oils and crude, cold-pressed, dark green pumpkinseed oil

- Crude wild oregano herb (as capsules with *Rhus coriaria*)

- Multiple spice complex (or extract), especially for muscular types with a history of diabetes; also helps strengthen the muscles

- Wild triple salt capsule with wild rosemary and oregano

- Wild kelp-based supplement with wild oregano and tyrosine, the kelp being derived from northern pacific and northern Atlantic sources

- Natural-source vitamin C, as a combination of camu camu, acerola, and rose hips

- Salt grass

Appendix B

Foods and supplements with hormone power, which influence the shape of the body and its metabolism.

Foods

- organic red meat
- organic poultry
- organic or grass-fed bison
- organic game
- organic lamb and mutton
- organic eggs
- organic whole milk
- organic cheese
- wild-source fish, especially fatty types
- wild-source seafood
- organic liver, kidney, and thymus

Supplements

- Undiluted 3x Royal Jelly
- Neroli Orange Blossom Water
- Damascene Rose Petal Water
- Wild Lavender Flower Water
- Wild Bay Leaf Water
- Wild Raw Bee Pollen
- Wild Raw Mountain Flower Honey

- Wild Raw Dandelion Honey
- Wild Raw Fir Tree Honey
- Wild Raw Oregano Honey
- Crude Austrian-Source Pumpkinseed Oil
- Crude Turkish-Source Sesame Seed Oil
- Wild Raw Kelp
- Extra Virgin Olive Oil
- Whole Raw Wild Red Palm Oil
- Raw Black Seed Oil
- Crude Steam-Extracted Wild Sockeye Salmon Oil
- Red Sour Grape Powder
- Emulsified Propolis
- Emulsified Wild Extract of Poplar Buds
- Raw Purple Maca Extract
- Raw Sarsaparilla Berry Extract
- Wild Chaga Mushroom Expresso
- Wild Chaga Mushroom Emulsified Drops

Appendix C

Fingernail signs of the different body types

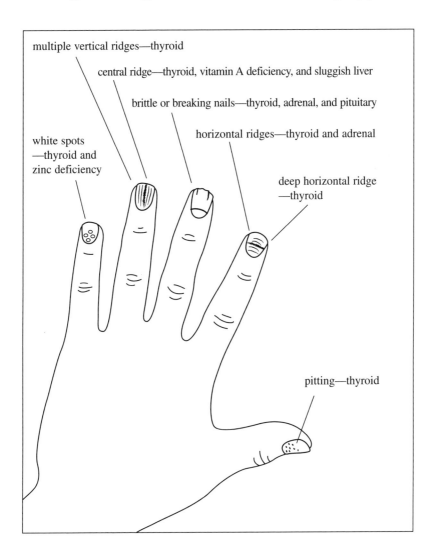

multiple vertical ridges—thyroid

central ridge—thyroid, vitamin A deficiency, and sluggish liver

brittle or breaking nails—thyroid, adrenal, and pituitary

horizontal ridges—thyroid and adrenal

white spots
—thyroid and
zinc deficiency

deep horizontal ridge
—thyroid

pitting—thyroid

Appendix D
Key characteristics of metabolic types

	thyroid	adrenal	pituitary	combination
head shape	square to rectangular	oval or narrow, head may be pointed	round and/or usually small for size of body	*
facial features	square chin, puffiness, jowls, thin upper lip	receding chin, crowding of lower teeth	pug or small nose, small mouth	*
body weight	front of thighs and abdomen	curvy buttocks, pouch below umbilicus	fat on sides of hips and heavily on buttocks	*
finger length	index finger is shorter than ring	index finger is longer than ring	about equal or index finger is slightly larger; short or small fingers	*
energy patterns	tired in the morning and more active at night	tired in the afternoon and evening	tired continuously	*
body temperature	low (may be cold all over), wears socks/sweaters to bed	low to normal (hands and feet often cold)	low to normal	*
body shape	apple	carrot, pouch below belly button	pear	*
hair pattern	coarse hair, male pattern baldness	fine or thin hair	fine to medium hair	*

* May be comprised of a combination of characteristics from thyroid, adrenal, and pituitary types

Bibliography

Anonymous. 1935. *Irish Country Recipes.*

Appenzeller, O. 1976. *The Autonomic Nervous System.* American Elsevier Publ. Co.

Barnes, B. 1976. *Hypothyroidism: The Unsuspected Illness.* New York: Harper-Collins.

Beiler, H. 1966. *Food is Your Best Medicine.* New York: Random House.

Benedict, E. *The Five Human Body Types.*

Best, C. H. and N. B. Taylor. 1945. *The Physiological Basis of Medical Practice.* Baltimore, MD: Williams & Wilkins Co.

Blaylock, R. 1997. *Excitotoxins.* Health Press.

Brown-Sequard, C. E. 1889. The effects produced in man by subcutaneous injection of a liquid obtained from testicles of animals. *Lancet.* 2:105-107.

Cott, Alan. *Fasting: The Ultimate Diet.* Hastings House.

Currier, W.D. 1969. Dizziness related to hypoglycemia: the role of adrenal steroids and nutrition. *J. Appl. Nutr.* 21(1&2).

D'Adamo, P. and C. Whitney. 2001. *Eat Right 4 Your Type.* New York: C. P. Putnam & Sons.

Daugherty, T. F. and A. White. 1944. Influence of hormones on lymphoid tissue structure and function. *Endocrinology.* 35:1.

DeGrout, L. 1979. *Endocrinology.* Grune & Stratton.

Goldman, H. B. and J. W. Tintera. 1956. Hypoadrenocorticism in otolaryngology. *AMA Archives of Otolaryngol.* 64:381.

Goldman, H. B. and J. W. Tintera. 1958. Stress and hypoadrenocorticism: the implications in otolaryngology. *Ann. Otol. Rhin. Laryn.* 67:185.

Greenblatt, R.B. 1945. *Office Endocrinology.* Springfield, IL: Charles C. Thomas.

Harrowa, H. 1932. *Practical Endocrinology.* Pioneer Printing Co.

Heim, C., et al. 2000. The potential role of hypocorticolism in the pathophysiology of stress-related bodily disorders. *Psychoneuroendocrinology.* (Jan).

Henkin, R. I. and D. H. Solomon. 1962. Salt-taste threshold in adrenal insufficiency in man. *J. Clin. Endocr.* 22:856.

Hill, N. (ed). 1994. *The Tomato Cookbook.* London: Reed International.

Ingram, C. 2005. *How to Eat Right and Live Longer.* Buffalo Grove, IL: Knowledge House Publishers.

Ingram, C. 2005. *The Cause for Cancer Revealed: the Vaccination Connection.* Buffalo Grove, IL: Knowledge House.

Ingram, C. 2006. *Nutrition Tests for Better Health.* Buffalo Grove, IL: Knowledge House Publishers.

Jennings, I. 1970. *Vitamins in Endocrine Metabolism.* William Heinemann Med. Books.

Kahn, Fritz. 1943. *Man in Structure and Function.* New York: Knopf.

Kelly, W. D. 1976. *The Metabolic Types.* Kelly Foundation.

Kretschner, Ern. 1925. *Physique and Character.* New York: Harcourt.

Lapin, J. H., Goldman, S. F., and A. Goldman. 1943. The clinical use of adrenal cortex hormones. *N. Y. State J. Med.* 43:1964.

Larson, T. H. 1929. *Why We Are What We Are: the Science and Art of Endocrine Therapy.* Chicago: American Endocrine Bureau.

Le Gross-Clark, W. E. 1946. *The Tissues of the Body.* Oxford: Oxford University Press.

Lucas, E. 1931. *Vegetable Cookery*. London: William Heinemann, Ltd.

Lust, J. B. 1962. *About Raw Juices: Their Therapeutic Value and Uses*. New York: Benedict Lust Publications.

Manohar, V., Ingram, C., Gray, J., et al. 2001. Antifungal activities of origanum oil against Candida albicans. *Molecular and Cellular Biochemistry*. 228:111-117.

McCarrison, Sir Robert. 1936. *Nutrition and National Health*. London: Faber and Faber.

McCollum, E. V. 1957. *A History of Nutrition: The Sequence of Ideas in Nutritional Investigation*. Boston: Houghton Mifflin Co.

Myer, J. H. and K. H. Schute. 1979. *Metabolic Aspects of Health*. Kentfield, CA: Discovery Press.

Perla, D. and J. Marmorston. 1935. Suprarenal corticol hormone and salt in the treatment of pneumonia and other severe infections. *The Eyes, Ears, Nose, and Throat Monthly*. 13:453.

Price, W. A. 1939. *Nutrition and Physical Degeneration*. Cancer Book House.

Rackemann, F. M. 1958. Asthma is a constitutional disease. *J. Allergy*. 29:535.

Roberts, S. E. 1967. *Exhaustion: Causes and Treatment*. Emmaus, PA: Rodale Books, Inc.

Senn, C. H. 1911. *How to Cook Vegetables*. Westminster: the Food and Cookery Development Agency.

Seyle, A. 1956. *The Stress of Life*. New York: McGraw-Hill.

Sheldon, W. H., Stevens, S. S. and W. B. Tucker. 1940. *Varieties of Human Physique: An Introduction to Constitutional Psychology*. Harper & Bros.

Shomon, M. J. 2004. *The Thyroid Diet*. New York: HarperCollins Publishers, Inc.

Siddiqui, Y. M., et al. 1996. Effect of essential oils on the enveloped viruses; antiviral activity of oregano oils on herpes simplex virus type 1 and Newcastle virus. *Medical Science Research*. 24:185.

Sinclair, H. M (ed). 1953. *The Work of Sir Robert McCarrison*. London: Faber and Faber.

Sivropoulou, A., et al. 1996. Antimicrobial and cytotoxic activities of Origanum essential oils. *J. Agric. Food Chem*. 44:1202.

Sugerman, A. A. and F. Haronian. 1994. Body type and sophistication of body concept. *J. Pers*. 32:380-394.

Talpur, N., Echard, B., Ingram, C., Bachi, D., and H. Preuss. 2001. Effects of a novel formulation of essential oils on glucose—insulin metabolism in diabetic and hypertensive rats: a pilot study. *Diabetes, Obesity, and Metabolism*. 7:193-199.

Tintera, J. W. 1955. The hypoadrenocortical state and its management. *N.Y. State J. Med*. 55(13).

Tintera, J. W. 1967. Endocrine aspects of schizophrenia: hypoglycemia of the hypoadrenocorticism. *J. Schizo*. 1:150.

Tintera, J. W. *Hypoadrenocorticism*. Mt. Vernon, New York: Adrenal Metabolic Research Society.

Tucker, L. A. 1984. Physical attractiveness, somatotype, and the male personality: a dynamic interactional perspective. *J. Clin. Psych*. 40:5, 1226.

Turner, C. D. 1948. *General Endocrinology. The Glands: Physiologic Specificity of Cortical Compounds*. Philadelphia: W.B. Saunders Co.

Tuttle, W. W. and B. A. Schottelius. 1969. *Textbook of Physiology*. St. Louis, MO: C.V. Mosby Co.

Williams, R.J. 1956. *Biochemical Individuality*. Austin: Univ. Texas Press.

Wolf, W. 1940. *Endocrinology in Modern Practice*. Philadelphia: W.B. Saunders Co.

Yesalis, C. E. and M. S. Bahrke. 2005. Anabolic steroid and stimulant use in North American Sport between 1850 and 1980. *Sport in History*. 25:434-451.

Index

thyroid-adrenal type and, 177, 179,
  359-360
thyroid type and, 105, 358, 379
Fingernails, 73, 104-106, 181, 215,
  227, 378
  brittle, 105, 378
  lack of moons, 106, 181
  ridges, 106, 378
  white spots on, 73, 105, 227, 378
Fluoride, 18, 266-268
  diseases and, 266
  sources of, 268
Food additives, 18, 33, 59, 174, 184,
  261, 272, 283-284
Food allergies, 25, 146, 184, 269-273
  see also Allergies
Food Intolerance Test, 270-271, 276
Fried Artichokes, 312-313
Fried Artichokes Au Parmesan, 313
Fried Cucumber, 313-314
Fried Organic or Grass-Fed Minute
  Steak, 330
Fried Wild Rice Topped with Organic
  Yogurt, 315
Fungal infections, 87, 104, 106, 125,
  137, 139, 280
Fungi, 53, 76, 86, 95, 104, 122, 126-128,
  163, 185-186, 204, 236, 279-282

G

Genetically engineered foods. *See*
  GMO
Gallbladder, 252, 269, 289
Glucagon, 45, 230
Gluten intolerance, 73, 227-228, 289
GMO, 17, 21, 33, 86, 99, 168, 198,

212, 251, 261-262, 273-274,
  277-278, 299
  soy, 17, 33, 86, 99, 212
Goiter, 93-94, 98-99, 243, 266
Goitrogens, 98-100, 297, 350
  sources of, 98-99, 100, 350
Grains, 25, 73, 100, 125, 160, 185-188,
  220, 224, 227-228, 231, 233, 248,
  289, 295, 298
  avoidance of, 185-186, 228
Grilled Fish Medley, 337
Grilled Marinated Wild Salmon with
  Pine Nuts, 329-330
Grilled Sour Prawns, 328
Gum Disease, 195, 198, 207

H

Hair, 45, 105-106, 115, 143-145, 156,
  177, 182-183, 2215, 231, 357-359,
  379
  brittle, 106
  coarse, 105, 358
  loss of, 105, 145, 231
  fine, 156, 359
Headaches, 19, 20, 72, 119, 1127, 140,
  155, 174, 176, 183, 201, 269, 271,
  273
  low blood sugar and, 72
  migraine, 140, 183, 269, 271
  treatment by type, 19, 20
Healthy Marzipan, 351
Heart disease, 9, 12, 15, 29, 45, 47,
  66, 71, 75, 86, 106, 192-193,
  195, 206-208, 218, 362, 364
  adrenal component, 71
  cholesterol and, 207-208

Lavender, 52, 59

Lecithin, 86, 249-253

Leukemia, 139, 223

Libido, 47, 50, 74

Liver, 39-40, 43, 49, 60, 62, 65-66, 69-71, 82, 135, 169-170, 205, 244, 250, 252, 275, 277, 289, 309, 313, 361-363
    food source, 69, 193, 234, 238, 251, 291, 332, 376

Lobster in Cream Sauce, 339

Low-Carb Vitamin-Rich Beef Stew, 339

Lupus, 9, 29, 139

Lyme disease, 9

Lymph, 29, 37, 52, 59, 249, 356, 362

Lymphoma, 223

Lysine, 247-249

M

Maca root, 29, 49, 140, 200, 238, 248, 299

Maca Root Adrenal Coffee, 344

Magnesium, 15, 98, 168, 199, 289, 373

Make-Your-Own-Salted Almonds, 342

Malnutrition, 259-264

Melatonin, 41, 241

Mental disorders, 17, 29, 41, 51, 72-73, 80, 82, 97, 115-120, 139, 141, 144-146, 201, 246, 255-259, 266, 269, 273, 363-364
    adrenals and, 51, 82, 115, 118-120, 139, 141, 256-257, 258, 363
    anger,17, 51, 120, 257
    anxiety, 17, 51, 72, 115, 118, 255, 258, 269
    glandular disorders and, 256-259, 363
    irritability, 41, 72, 115, 201, 257, 273
    manic-depressive disorder, 256, 258
    panic attacks, 17, 72, 118, 141, 144-145, 255-258
    poor concentration, 97, 115, 146, 256
    schizophrenia, 256
    see also Depression; Stress

Mercury, 153, 159, 162-163, 210-211, 213, 297, 309, 329
    pituitary gland and, 162

Mesomorphs, 21

Metabolic disorders, 8, 9, 14-15, 31

Metabolic Salad, 308-309

Metabolism, 7, 9, 14, 20, 23-37, 42, 63-70, 75-84, 163, 169, 185, 189, 197, 207, 215, 239, 247-248, 255, 285-289, 294, 297, 356, 364
    body shape and, 35
    climate and, 36
    thyroid hormone and, 64-70
    weight gain and, 31, 37, 65, 297

Milk, 98-99, 134, 167, 191, 197-200, 222, 224-225, 229, 232-234, 237, 275-279, 290
    allergy, 167, 199, 275-276
    toxins in, 198, 277-279

Mixed Berries in Whole Fat Milk, 349

Monsanto, 101, 281–282

Mostly Adrenal Smoothie, 345-346

MSG, 17, 261, 270, 272, 282-283

Multiple Sclerosis, 202,234